**Michael Grose** is one of Australia's leading parenting and educational writers and speakers. He is the author of ten books for parents, including the bestselling *Why First-Borns Rule the World*. Currently he supports more than 100( Australia and internationally to build strong partn communities.

**Dr Jodi Richardson** is a wellbeing ex who specialises in helping parents a more relaxed, resilient and optimistic kids with flourishing mental health. She combines nine years of university study with over twenty years of professional work in wellbeing, clinical practice, elite sport and education in all that she shares. She's a mum of two and travels extensively speaking to parents and schools.

# Anxious Kids

# Michael Grose
# & Dr Jodi Richardson

LIFE

*The information contained in this book is for general purposes only.*
*It is not intended as and should not be relied upon as medical advice.*
*A medical practitioner should be consulted if you have any concerns*
*about you, or your child's, mental health.*

Penguin Life

UK | USA | Canada | Australia
India | New Zealand | South Africa | China

Penguin Books is part of the Penguin Random House group of companies
whose addresses can be found at global.penguinrandomhouse.com.

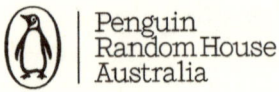

Penguin
Random House
Australia

First published by Penguin Random House Australia Pty Ltd 2019

Text copyright © Michael Grose and Jodi Richardson 2019

The moral right of the authors has been asserted.

Cover design by James Rendall © Penguin Random House Australia Pty Ltd
Cover figures by sattva78/Shutterstock and Rawpixel.com/Shutterstock
Typeset in 12/16 pt Berkeley by Midland Typesetters, Australia
Printed and bound in Australia by Griffin Press, an accredited ISO AS/NZ 14001
Environmental Management Systems printer.

A catalogue record for this
book is available from the
National Library of Australia

ISBN 978 0 14379 495 0

penguin.com.au

Michael:
*For Astrid, Max, Ruby, Harry and Grace.*

Jodi:
*To Peter, I treasure our love and our life together.*
*To Hunter and Mackinley, who fill me with joy,*
*and to my parents, Cheryl and Rick, and brother Adam*
*for a lifetime of love, support and encouragement.*

# Contents

# Introduction

You are about to make a big difference in the life of your anxious child. As you read on what these changes involve will become more apparent to you, but for now, let us simply tell you that the understanding, knowledge and strategies you'll learn here, and apply in your family, will make a profound difference to your child's life, now and over their lifetime.

Children who experience anxiety feel different. Sometimes they think they're broken. Of course, we know they're not. Far from it. They can also feel very alone and think that no one will ever be able to understand what they're going through, let alone help them. Understanding that anxiety is a well understood and manageable condition brings anxious kids such relief. We hope that just by reading that you breathed a sigh of relief too, and your shoulders dropped a little further away from your ears. Because what we do know is that anxiety often runs in families. So it's possible you, or your child's other parent, know anxiety all too well. And there's little that increases the anxiety of parents more than perceiving their kids are struggling. Especially when they're struggling with their mental health.

We understand. This is personal. We've both experienced anxiety for as long as we can remember. We know what it's like to be the anxious kid who worries about everything, who can't always breathe properly, who jumps at shadows and knows something's not right but has no idea what to do about it. We both grew up with at least one parent who was anxious and who had never even heard of anxiety as a condition, let alone understood it, or knew how to help themselves, or us as kids.

We've written this book so that you have the understanding our parents never did. So that you can recognise anxiety in your child*, and help them to understand and manage their anxiety in a way that moves it from centre stage to background noise.

Anxiety doesn't have to be a shadow that clouds the days of children and teenagers. As you share with them what you learn as you read on, in age-appropriate ways (we help you with that too), you'll feel less anxious and more confident to play a key role in supporting your child or teen, to give them the gift of understanding themselves and to skill them up to observe anxiety as background noise that they can notice and accept, before turning their attention to what really matters – living life in full colour.

---

\* Throughout the book we write about 'children', 'your child' and 'kids'. These references encompass children in families and classrooms from pre-school age through to eighteen years.

# Part 1

# Anxiety is a problem

As the parent of an anxious child, you're most certainly not alone. Millions of families all over the world are right there with you. Though it's helpful to know, we understand that it doesn't make the challenging role of parenting an anxious child any easier. What will is developing and deepening your understanding of childhood anxiety and the important role you play in helping them manage it.

As part of a family, the impact of a child's anxiety is felt by the child, their parents and their siblings. It's natural to feel frustrated, saddened, worried and unsure when you're parenting an anxious child. There are times when a child's anxiety impacts on the family in ways that are hard to manage. From the kids being late to school or not wanting to go at all, to parents not making it to work or being unable to get much done because they are so worried, it can be disruptive to the point of exasperation and exhaustion.

This section of the book will help you begin to understand anxiety on a deeper level. You'll learn how common it really is, factors that contribute to it, how it can be mistaken or misunderstood, why it won't go away on its own, how your family has come to choreograph its very own anxiety dance, and much more.

We're taking this journey with you. We're in this together. Step by step your knowledge will grow and with that you'll feel more empowered with each passing chapter to support your child in ways that are productive, helpful and enable them to move towards living a rich and full life.

# 1

# The anxiety epidemic

## First things first

The future has never been so bright for anxious kids. The mental health landscape, which once was dry and barren, is now green and filled with hope and the promise of recognition; of understanding, of acceptance, empathy and compassion; and rich in resources, support and help.

While parenting an anxious child can feel overwhelming and difficult at first, we want you to think about it differently. We want you to take a moment to recognise that you, your anxious child and your family have been presented with an opportunity.

To be anxious is to be human. Everybody experiences it. It can be a temporary experience under stressful circumstances or it can be a thread through the fabric of who we are. Over a lifetime, one in four adults will experience an anxiety disorder. Of those, half will have their first symptoms by the time they're fifteen years old.[1] Many go undiagnosed for years. If you too have anxiety, there's every chance it went undetected for far too long. That was certainly the case for us.

Noticing that your child is showing signs or symptoms of anxiety is a gift to them. We can't change what is happening right in front of us, and we can't undo it. What will help your anxious child to flourish, despite their anxiety, is first and foremost someone recognising they need help.

From that point forward, anxious children can get the under-standing, support, skills, strategies and, if needs be, the treatment that will help them to manage their anxiety now and over the course of their life. It's not a diagnosis that needs to sap you or your child of the hope for a vibrant, meaningful and fulfilling life. It's a treatable mental health condition, and the sooner addressed the better.

## Beginning to understand anxiety

Anxiety triggers part of the brain to fire up the fight-or-flight response or, as some aptly call it, the fight, flight, freeze or freak-out response,[2] to protect us from danger. It's an emotion, and like other emotions it has a start, a middle and an end.

Except anxiety doesn't end for some.

That's the experience for an estimated half a million plus Australian kids and 117 million worldwide who have an anxiety disorder.[3] That's how far-reaching and common anxiety has become.

For these kids, their experience of anxiety doesn't end when the threat, danger or stressful situation has passed. The anxiety they experience can disrupt their day-to-day life and family life in both predictable and unexpected ways. Anxiety has the potential to stand in the way of kids being kids and their ability to enjoy the quintessential elements of a happy, relaxed, carefree, playful childhood; but it doesn't have to.

Anxious kids have a brain that works really hard to protect them from danger. A part of their brain is similar to the sentinel among meerkats who is always on its tippy-toes watchfully assess-ing the environment for threats. This means that anxious kids spend an inordinate amount of time with their fight-or-flight response in full swing.

It's not by choice. It's exhausting, and not just for the kids. Whether the threat is real or imagined, the brain and body react in the same way. An oversensitive brain will protect, protect, protect, even if the 'threat' seems innocuous to everybody else, or possibly isn't even noticeable. Once the senses signal to the brain that danger is apparent, it's comparable to opening the floodgates. The anxiety cascade begins as does the fallout, making a hard job more challenging for parents of an anxious child.

## #worldstoughestjob

In 2015 a job ad was placed online and in newspapers by US greeting card company American Greetings. As interviews were held for the 'director of operations' role, more details about the position came to light. It was revealed that the role was physically demanding, with an expectation the director would be on their feet most of the time. In fact, the requirement was that the director could be active from 135 to an unlimited number of hours a week. Other qualities important for the role included excellent negotiation and interpersonal skills, a degree in medicine, a degree in finance and a degree in the culinary arts. The environment in which the director would work was described as chaotic, and work would often be undertaken without a break. If the director wanted lunch, they would have to wait until their associates had eaten first. The interviewer also explained that if applicants had a life, they'd be asked to give it up. There were no vacations provided and when holidays came around, such as Christmas and Thanksgiving, there was no downtime; in fact, the workload would increase. The position was twenty-four hours a day, seven days a week, 365 days a year. All with no pay.

The video recording of the interviews went viral, amassing over 27 million views to date. The applicants' reactions were priceless when they found out the job ad was fake and was indeed describing the role of mothers all over the world as part of American Greetings' clever #worldstoughestjob marketing campaign for Mother's Day. Of course, dads are equally important in children's lives.

There's no denying parenting is a tough gig. It's also exhilarating, emotional, heart-warming, demanding, wonderful, exhausting, meaningful, frustrating, heart-wrenching, awe-inspiring and incredibly fulfilling. It's the most important and profound 'job' any of us will ever do. It's as different as it is the same for all of us; there's no operations manual and we never quite know what each day is going to bring. When our kids are struggling, it tears at our hearts in ways we could never prepare ourselves for.

## Our job isn't to protect them, not from everything

Witnessing the suffering of our children is a difficult burden to bear, no matter how old they are. It's helpful if we remind ourselves as parents that our role isn't to protect our kids from life's hardships, but to steer and guide them, and to help them get back up again when life knocks them down. Remembering this is as much for our own sanity as it is for their resilience.

To continue the metaphor: anxiety is one of life's knocks that kids can get back up from. Our role as parents in helping them do just that can never be underestimated. They learn so much from us that builds their confidence and resilience, and helps them handle anxiety when it crops up or creeps in. Lifestyle choices, thinking skills, coping strategies, values, play, self-care, compassion, empathy, gratitude, relationships, kindness and an ability to see the bigger picture in life all play a part in helping them to manage their anxiety.

These are just some of the impactful ways our teaching and role modelling help our children to move anxiety from centre stage. You can help them. You are helping them. As you learn more about anxiety, where it comes from and how to help your child manage it, you'll be integral to their flourishing.

## Just how common is anxiety?

Parents all over the world are dealing with anxious children. Between the tender age of four and the brink of adulthood at seventeen, on average one in seven kids are diagnosed with a mental illness in Australia.[4]

Of all those kids, half are diagnosed with an anxiety disorder. That equates to roughly two kids in every Australian classroom, though some, if separation anxiety is in play, often don't even make it to school. Anxiety disorders are the top disease burden for females aged between five and forty-four. For boys and young men the top disease burdens are suicide and self-harm.[5] These boys and young men are integral to the data but their experiences are far from academic. Most don't understand why they think and feel the way they do and why they're suffering. Many feel broken, and it impacts on the entire family unit.

When Australia conducted the first Child and Adolescent Survey of Mental Health and Wellbeing in 1998, anxiety disorders weren't included. It wasn't on the radar in the same way major depressive disorder and attention deficit hyperactivity disorder (ADHD) were. It's fair to say it's on the radar now.

The second and most recent Australian Child and Adolescent Survey of Mental Health and Wellbeing, published in 2015, paints a picture of the state of mental health of Aussie kids. It's no oil painting.

Kids with a diagnosis of an anxiety disorder included those experiencing separation anxiety, social phobia, generalised anxiety disorder or obsessive-compulsive disorder. Anxiety disorders such as specific phobias – spiders, for example, or panic disorder or agoraphobia – weren't caught in the research net. Many anxious kids also go undetected. We think it's reasonable, prudent in fact, to suggest that current statistics underestimate the enormity of the problem.

## How has children's anxiety changed?

Professor Jean Twenge from San Diego State University is a researcher dedicated to understanding changes in youth mental health over generations. Professor Twenge and her colleagues crunched the numbers on mental illness data from over 77 000 American college and high school students between 1938 and 2007. Between the 1930s and 1940s an average of 50 out of 100 students scored above average on measures of mental disorders. That number has now jumped to 85 out of every 100. That's a 70 per cent increase in the number of students with symptoms of mental illness.[6]

Similar research looking specifically at anxiety showed that the average American child in the 1980s reported more anxiety than child psychiatric patients in the 1950s.[7] Increases in anxiety across generations have also been identified in China and the UK.[8]

Kids are in the thick of an anxiety epidemic, and the role of parents is crucial.

Staggering as the numbers are, the stats don't tell the whole story. Each and every child enveloped by a statistic is a person – a young person whose life has taken a turn in an unexpected direction.

## Anxiety misunderstood

The breadth and depth of an anxious kid's struggle is often mis-understood and, at times, unrecognised. Parents are presenting at hospitals worried about their kids, not recognising that the symptoms they're witnessing are, in fact, symptoms of mental illness.

This is precisely what was revealed by Aisha Dow in her health feature 'The Worrying Mental Health Trend Affecting Australians' in *The Age*. In the article, Professor Harriet Hiscock from the Murdoch Children's Research Institute in Melbourne said parents were bringing their children to hospital without realising they were experiencing anxiety or depression. 'They thought the panic attacks were seizures, or the recurrent tummy aches were a physical problem, when really it was anxiety.'

Professor Hiscock and her team analysed the number of visits to Victorian emergency departments by under twenty-year-olds over seven years and found a 46 per cent increase in the number of kids and teenagers seeking help for stress-related disorders, mainly anxiety.[9]

## Anxiety has many faces

Kids experience anxiety in different ways. Some anxious kids can appear happy most of the time, but struggle with anxiety that affects only parts of their life, or shows up intermittently. Others can endure any one or a combination of frightening thoughts, inexplicable fear or dread, unrealistic to catastrophic worries, and physical symptoms varying from tummy aches to dizziness to not being able to get a full breath, to spotty vision.

In the early days anxiety is easy to overlook, often mistaken for blips in behaviour, attention, confidence, resilience and physical health. Your little one doesn't want to play at the park with the other kids? He's a little shy. Your primary schooler has a meltdown when you visit the shopping centre? She's just tired and having another tantrum. Fourth grader feeling too sick to go to school? Could be that food intolerance playing up again. Teenager won't sit still and can't concentrate in class? She's fidgety and disruptive.

There are parents everywhere doing their best to raise their kids and help them navigate their shyness, tantrums and tendency to fidget. Nothing to see here. Just another day in the life of parents. Then there are the kids who struggle to socialise or spend even a moment in big open spaces with crowds of people, or who become nauseated from worry about separating from their mum or dad.

These kids also struggle to concentrate because they're constantly in fight-or-flight mode.

Developmentally appropriate fears, worries and reactions to stress, paired with behaviour, personality, temperament, environment, circumstances and parenting combine in ways that can make it tricky for us as parents to recognise when our kids might in fact be beginning to battle with anxiety and in need of some extra help.

If there's even a fleeting possibility that this is your child, make an appointment with your GP to ask some questions. Some of the common symptoms of anxiety, such as an upset tummy, could indeed be related to a physical cause with a simple explanation.

## It won't go away on its own

When anxiety goes unrecognised it goes untreated, and when it goes untreated it typically gets worse over time, not better. Anxiety presents in a range of ways in different children – worry being a common feature. Understandably, worrying makes it hard to concentrate. Anxious kids often reflect on past events or anticipate what's to come; their minds are regularly anywhere but in the moment. It's no surprise it impacts learning.

Anxious kids struggle more with reading, and academically in general.[10] It's also well understood that those experiencing anxiety as children are at higher risk of experiencing major depression and an anxiety disorder as adults.[11]

If you're one of the one in four adults experiencing an anxiety disorder, it's possible that you're just beginning to realise it now, or maybe you can't remember a life where you weren't anxious. It turns out that anxiety starts to show up much earlier than other mental illnesses but can be easily overlooked.[12]

While it won't go away of its own accord, anxiety is a deeply researched, well understood and treatable condition.

## Liang's story

Liang remembers times throughout her childhood where she was completely overwhelmed by her anxiety. She loved netball and played at quite a high level from a young age. By the time she was sixteen she was playing A-grade netball with and against women twice her age. She found that time in her netball career to be both brilliant and stressful. Liang always put more pressure on herself than anyone else ever did. She started to have trouble breathing during games. She couldn't seem to fill her lungs. Her parents took her to see the doctor where the anxiety she was experiencing was mistaken for asthma. She was prescribed Ventolin to help.

Signs and symptoms of anxiety disorders, many overlapping, can be fleeting and are developmentally normal experiences for most kids. It's not surprising that anxiety in kids can go undetected for months, years or, in some cases, decades. It's easy to see from Liang's story that anxiety could be overlooked or mistaken for other problems.

## Why is it hard to recognise?

There are many reasons anxiety goes undetected in kids; unlike a sore foot, a jammed finger or a cold, it's not an obvious ailment. Anxiety is internal. The nature of it means it can be hard for a parent to notice their child is struggling. That is, of course, unless your child is firstly able to recognise their fears and worries (and not just be consumed by them) and is then able to share them with you.

Noticing the content of thoughts is an important life skill. It's something we do as adults every day. But, ironically, we may not notice. If you stop to think about it (no pun intended), we reflect on our thoughts and knowledge all the time. Every time we reach for our phones to look up an answer to a question, we do so because we know we don't know.

## Thought-noticing

The scientific term for noticing what you're thinking is called metacognition, often described as 'thinking about thinking'. It's a unique skill we have as humans and takes our thinking beyond what we learn and know, to reflecting on the content of our thinking. It's a critical skill to hone in anxious kids.

Thoughts can have an unwieldly power over all of us, especially kids who haven't yet developed the skilfulness to notice the content of their thoughts.

It's common for gorgeous little three-year-olds (aka threenagers) to tantrum like it's going out of fashion. The part of the brain responsible for emotional regulation is yet to mature. Despite this, amazing changes are happening in other parts of their brains. This is in fact the age that some kids show the first roots of metacognition but there's still a way to go.[13]

Professor John H Flavell from Stanford University is considered the guru when it comes to understanding the development of kids' ability to think about their thinking. In one study he asked five-year-olds, eight-year-olds and adults to think of something they enjoyed doing and something they didn't enjoy, and then to say their specific thoughts while they were thinking. The adults and eight-year-olds were able to comply, but only some of the five-year-olds were able to do this task.[14]

Children develop the ability to notice and share the content of their thoughts between around Grade Two and early high school.[15] The importance of this developmental change for anxious kids is huge. A listening ear and an empathetic response is what anxious kids need in order to feel comfortable sharing their thoughts with someone they trust. It's usually mothers they turn to. Kids can have worries or might even describe the thoughts they're having as 'bad'. It's not a big jump from having a bad thought to feeling like a bad person for some kids.

Noticing is just the first part; having the thinking skills to be able to handle difficult thoughts comes later and doesn't rely on having more control. We will look in greater detail later in this book at how you can use thought-noticing as a tool for managing your child's anxiety in positive ways.

## Thought control – fact or fiction?

Control is comforting, isn't it? The ability to control what we think and feel is enticing, but it's not possible – not for long, anyway. Most of us grow up to believe that we have more control over our thoughts than we do. Trying not to think about something is the surest way to keep it front of mind. After all, the brain has to remember what it's not allowed to think about!

Stanford University guru Professor Flavell conducted other studies to get a clearer understanding of when kids realise they don't actually have much control over what they think. This happens around eight years of age.[16] By the time they're around thirteen years old most kids know that thoughts can come and go whether they like them or not, and that they don't always have a say over the content of their thoughts.

## Why 'Don't worry about it' doesn't help

Anxious kids often hear, 'Don't worry about it.' Kids with worries seek reassurance from parents all the time. The constant need for reassurance is a hallmark of anxiety. Anxious kids just want to be told everything is going to be okay. It's natural, of course, for a parent to want to reassure their anxious child that there's no monster under the bed, they'll ace the test or that going away on school camp will be brilliant. Unfortunately, and you probably know this from experience, it doesn't help. Any suggestion of

'Don't worry, you'll be fine' is asking for the child to control their thinking, which we know they can't do. None of us can.

Constant worrying is so hard for little ones to cope with, and no wonder they turn to their parents to affirm that they're going to be okay. It lifts the weight of the world off their shoulders, but not for long. Unfortunately, their anxious minds are soon worrying about something else, and the need for reassurance comes back.

## The Anxiety Dance

Inevitably, this becomes a cycle which child and adolescent psychologist Dr Chris McCurry calls the 'Anxiety Dance'. He explains it beautifully with his ABCD model. It's the culmination of three main 'moves': the 'activator', 'behaviour' and 'consequences'.

A  Activator
B  Behaviour
C  Consequences
D  Dance

### Activator

The challenging event for the child is the activator. You could also call this the triggering event. The activator for a child experiencing separation anxiety could be saying goodbye to their parent outside their classroom at the start of a school day.

### Behaviour

Behaviour is how the child expresses their anxiety. These are all of the signs you'll see that your child is feeling anxious – the outward expression of what they're feeling. Behaviour might be in the form of tears, refusal to say goodbye, clinging and an upset stomach for the child who can't bear to part with their parent.

## Consequences

The consequences come next, and this is all about how you as a parent think and feel. It's common for parents of anxious kids to feel worried, upset, anxious, frustrated, angry or any combination of these and more. It's also common to have thoughts that can be distressing or guilt-laden: 'This won't ever end', 'It's embarrassing', 'Why does everyone else's child manage but not mine' or 'I just can't keep doing this every day'.

## Putting it all together

Next comes the dance, which is doing anything necessary to end the anxiety for your child by removing the challenge. In the case of the child who feels extremely upset about separating at the classroom door, the dance could include a parent picking up their child, reassuring them with loads of cuddles and then taking them home to end the distress. This dance soon becomes a pattern.

The child learns that their desperate need to stop feeling anxious can be achieved with their parents' help. Avoiding their activator helps anxious kids minimise their distress. The more an anxious child practises avoidance, the harder it will be for them to manage their anxiety and move forward to do what's important, such as saying goodbye to their mum or dad and going to school.

With each instance of avoidance, the pattern perpetuates and the anxiety strengthens. It's a perfectly understandable need under the circumstances.

This is the anxiety dance. It relieves anxiety in the short term, but doesn't help the child to develop the skills to manage their anxiety. The answer always falls on eliminating any distress.

Reassurance in the manner of 'Don't worry about it' or 'Don't think about it' becomes a part of the dance. All the while, loving parents temporarily minimise the distress of their child (and their own, which can often be much needed), while reinforcing an unhelpful series of dance steps.

This is a common approach by concerned parents, as only around half of adults understand that it's impossible to *not think*.[17] Asking anxious kids to 'not worry about it' isn't the answer. While we're awake, our minds generate a continuous flow of content known as a 'stream of consciousness'.

So if *not thinking* is impossible, what's the alternative?

## Looking at thoughts, not from them

A powerful way to help kids to manage anxiety is to encourage them to look at, rather than from, difficult thoughts. This concept was coined by Professor Stephen Hayes, a much published, highly respected psychologist and the developer of Acceptance and Commitment Therapy, a widely used evidence-based therapy for the treatment of anxiety and other psychological conditions.

When anxious kids look through their thoughts it's as if they're being pulled down a river by a strong current. The ability of anxious kids to notice and recognise their intrusive and difficult thoughts is akin to standing on the riverbank and watching the river flow by.

With these skills kids can let us know as parents that they're not coping with the content of their thoughts, and we can recognise their need for help.

Thank goodness our thoughts are private. We all have thoughts that can go against the grain of who we are, or are so irrational that explaining them would be embarrassing. These thoughts can be judgemental, blaming or unkind, fleeting as they may be.

As adults, we learn that thoughts aren't always facts and we dismiss them without realising we're doing so. When kids are anxious, their thoughts can hang around, giving them another reason to worry. 'Why am I thinking this?' 'I don't want to think this way but I can't stop.' 'What's wrong with me?' 'What would people think of me if only they knew what I think about?' 'What will Mum or Dad think of me if I tell them?'

Anxious kids can feel ashamed of their thoughts. The content of their thoughts can confuse and embarrass them so they refuse to say them out loud – more so as they approach or enter their teenage years. Strange and scary thoughts can be hard to share, even with their most trusted confidante.

## Telling them isn't enough – we need to show them

Worries and painful or difficult thoughts are part of the anxiety puzzle for many kids, but not all. They need someone to talk with. We can tell our kids we're there for them, but our words aren't enough. We have to show them.

Kids spell love as T-I-M-E. The concept is a bit corny, but true. A loving, nurturing relationship with our kids, built through spending quality time together, helps them to feel comfortable sharing their thoughts with us.

Show them love by being present in between the times they need us, as well as when they're in need of our support. By stopping what we're doing, putting down the phone, the vegetable peeler, the work, by making eye contact and being present. If we do this, we earn their trust by showing them we're available. They won't come to us if they feel they're always interrupting something or that other tasks are more important to us. Being present with our kids is the most important time we'll spend as parents.

## The sooner we know, the sooner we can help

Anxiety can be overlooked for many reasons. Often day-to-day functioning of anxious kids won't be affected in obvious ways and they can generally be happy. It won't necessarily consume their every waking moment, but there will be signs of anxiety if you know what to look for.

Early detection is critical. Recognising anxiety in kids is the first job. Even knowing that what they're going through has a name and other kids are going through the same challenge can bring relief, notwithstanding the fact that recognition is the first step towards help. They feel heard, understood and optimistic. That's an excellent start.

## Anxiety is contagious

You know those last-minute requests that can pop up just as you're leaving for school in the morning? The hair is brushed, teeth are cleaned, bags are packed, shoes are on and even the car is warming up, if it's cold, then comes, 'Can you please sign my homework book?', 'I forgot to empty the dishwasher', 'I left my shoes in the rain and they're wet' or 'I owe Jack five dollars, he bought lunch for me yesterday'.

Bell time is looming.

Your hopes of getting to work or an appointment on time are fading.

Your stress level rises, anxiety builds and everyone feels it.

Stress and anxiety are contagious. Kids 'catch' it from us and we can 'catch' it from them.

## How is anxiety contagious?

Keen to understand more about how this happens, one group of researchers, led by Wendy Mendes from the University of California, devised a fascinating experiment to measure if stress experienced by a mother is 'caught' by her infant.

Each mum in the study took a friend or relative and their 12–14-month-old baby along to the experiment. Whenever the baby wasn't with their mum, they were with someone they knew, trusted and felt relaxed with.

At the beginning of the experiment each mother and her baby enjoyed time together so they were both feeling comfortable and relaxed. The researcher took stress-related measurements as a baseline while the mothers were feeling comfortable and content. The mothers then completed a questionnaire. The experiment began and the mothers' stress levels were continuously monitored.

One at a time, each mother in the experiment performed exactly the same task, which included giving a five-minute speech in front of two evaluators detailing her strengths and weaknesses. After each speech the evaluators had five minutes to ask each mum questions.

Picture this. You've just given your five-minute speech about your strengths and weaknesses to two strangers and now you're answering their questions. The evaluators are nodding, smiling and leaning forward.

You feel good, don't you? This is positive feedback. You know they're enjoying listening to you and approving of your answers, and you're reassured you're doing a good job.

This was the experience for some of the mothers; for others it wasn't quite so good.

The parents who agreed to take part in the research were divided into three groups. One group received positive feedback, one group wasn't asked questions by the evaluators but simply answered a few questions alone, and the third group received negative feedback. As they gave their speech to the evaluators and answered their questions, the evaluators became progressively more negative by frowning, shaking their heads, crossing their arms and leaning back.

After their speech and question-and-answer session, each mother completed another questionnaire and was reunited with her baby. No prizes for guessing which group of mums experienced the most stress! Giving a speech to strangers about yourself is stressful enough without being on the receiving end of frowning and negative body language.

It was fascinating that the infants were immediately affected by their mothers' stress. Even though the infants were never exposed to any stress directly, they picked up their mothers' anxieties.

Stress in the children, measured via heart-rate changes, instantaneously mirrored that of their stressed parents. The research team speculate that a mother's stress was communicated to her baby by her facial expressions, posture, touch, voice tone and patterns and odour.[18] Fascinating!

## It all makes sense now

Do you remember what it was like trying to settle a crying baby when you were tired and stressed? As parents we tried to act calm on the outside but our insides would be churning and we would be pleading, 'Please just go to sleep.' These monologues may or may not have been G rated! The more stressed we became the more we felt the need for our babies to settle, and the less they would. Our stress was contagious. No wonder they got so wound up!

When you're running on barely any sleep and every second of the day is spent parenting full throttle with kids, it can be hard. We're not telling you anything new. There are times when we can speak impatiently to our kids, overreact or even yell at them. At these times we're usually dealing with our own anxiety as well as upset kids.

### Imari's story

When Imari was in prep he had two stressed teachers. They yelled all the time. Not at him directly, just the general kind of constant yelling thrown around a classroom that, eventually, everybody takes on board. Imari ended up with tummy aches and didn't want to go to school. His teachers' stress and anxiety upset him terribly. He was only four.

He complained of tummy aches every day but was still sent to school. His mum and dad knew he wasn't sick. Not physically anyway. Imari's appetite was good, he didn't have a fever and wasn't vomiting. Until one day when he did: all over the kid in front of him as the class sat cross-legged on the floor while their teachers marked the roll. His daily complaints about feeling sick and not wanting to go to school were always brushed aside and the time Imari was genuinely ill, no one believed him.

Students in classrooms with stressed teachers have elevated levels of the stress hormone cortisol.[19] Kids who are anxious, like Imari, find these environments stressful as they easily 'catch' the anxiety of their teachers.

When you're running late for school and work, the anxiety that rises is often temporary. This is the regular human emotion we all know. The stressor – not being on time in that case – is inter-preted as a danger by our brain. Suddenly, we're on high alert and the fight-or-flight response kicks in. When all's said and done, when we're eventually on our way and the kids realise that there'll be no need for a late pass, everyone relaxes and the anxiety passes. But for people with an anxiety disorder, the anxiety hangs around long after the party's over.

An understanding that anxiety is contagious is powerful. Especially when we're at home with our own families, where we feel most comfortable and we're more likely to let our guard down. Inside our own four walls our feelings are more likely to spill over from what's considered 'socially acceptable'. In private we can rejoice and sing and dance in ridiculous ways when we're excited, and cry when we're devastated. We're more prone to taking the lid off our stress and anxiety at home to let off psychological steam. Our homes are places we can safely feel and express our feelings but we also need to regulate our emotions in ways that, firstly, don't spread our stress and anxiety to kids and, secondly, teach them to handle their emotions in healthy ways.

## Jodi's story

If I'm out and about and feeling anxious, most of the time I'll recognise and manage it in the moment. It's unlikely anyone else would know. Anxious people are good like that – one of the many faces of anxiety is the mask that goes on and off depending on the circumstances. I talk openly about my anxiety with friends and family, and even when speaking to audiences during a presentation, but I know that the fella behind the register at Woolies doesn't need (or want!) to know.

When I'm at home, I can be more open and seek the help, comfort and support I need. We can all learn and gain much from knowing how each other is feeling. We want our kids to share with us their emotional 'temperature' and to learn the language of emotional literacy beyond feeling 'good', 'sad' or 'scared'. As parents, we can teach our kids to not be afraid of emotions when we share our own and talk openly about how we're managing them.

My kids know I have an anxiety disorder. I talk openly about it often. Most of the time it's background noise; I've learned how to turn the dial right down. There are, of course, times when stress of the 'ordinary' variety gets the better of me and starts to impact my mood, my patience and how I respond.

When that's happening I practise coping out loud, or failing to cope out loud as is sometimes the case. I learned this technique from Seattle-based child and adolescent psychologist Dr Chris McCurry. During an interview for an online course, Dr McCurry talked at length about the many strategies parents can practise to help anxious kids. He talked about coping out loud as a way of demonstrating to kids the thinking and decision-making behind our choices as parents when we're struggling emotionally. It's like pulling back the curtain on our minds so our kids can see the cogs turning as we unveil our thoughts, how we feel about them and what we're doing, or going to do, about them.

'See me, you guys? This is me taking some long, slow, deep breaths because I'm feeling frustrated/anxious right now.' This is what I've been known to say if my kids are squabbling or needing one too many reminders to get moving or finish a task. I'll say something similar to that when I feel my emotional temperature climbing. Most of the time. Other times I might tell them I'm simply feeling anxious for no reason and that they'll notice I'm not my usual happy, cheerful and relaxed self. I tell them that I'm okay, that I'm practising acceptance of how I'm feeling, it's nothing they've done and that it will pass. My anxiety is well managed, so those scenarios don't come up often. I flourish despite my anxiety. Your kids can too.

It's an emotional heads-up and it makes a genuine difference to how everyone feels and acts. Kids can feel responsible when their parents aren't happy; it's important they know they're not (if they're not!).

## It goes both ways

On the flip side, it's equally imperative to be mindful that kids' anxieties, worries and stresses are contagious. Our instinct as parents is to nurture and protect our kids. When they come to us feeling overwhelmed, wound up or anxious, we can easily feel the same way they do. That's what's meant to happen, to a point.

Our children turn to us and communicate how they're feeling in ways that evoke an emotional response within us. This is an evolutionary ploy to kindle our empathy so we feel how they feel and are highly motivated to help. It's easy, though, to be swept up in the emotion, to become anxious ourselves and to react in ways that can make matters worse.

## Matching our emotional response

There's a lovely middle ground. Showing what's called a 'matched' emotional response is a way to demonstrate to our kids that we understand them. We can do this by matching our facial expressions, posture, tone of voice and body language to theirs.

Have you ever felt devastated, angry or even enraged, only to be 'comforted' by someone who is as Zen as a Buddhist monk? It makes you feel like they simply don't get it.

When matching emotions we start where they are, and then little by little bring our emotions down a few pegs at a time. When we're connected with each other, and take our time, they'll follow suit and will soon begin to settle down.

The contagious nature of anxiety spreads equally from child to parent as it does from parent to child. Our discomfort at our children's crying, stress or worry can prompt us to want to shut it down quickly because of the distress it causes us.

By noticing anxiety in your child, and by demonstrating a willingness to sit with them in their distress, you're teaching them to do the same. An acceptance of emotions in the present moment, without needing to fix the problem or cheer them up, is counterintuitive but revolutionary. The ability to tolerate discomfort is within all of us – it's just not something we're good at. We want problems solved and uncomfortable feelings gone. Now. Remarkably, as we teach our children to recognise, understand and label how they feel, and support them as they say to themselves or aloud 'I'm feeling anxious', the emotion can begin to lose some of its stranglehold. It's the running away from anxiety that amplifies it. When our kids learn to stop, turn around and face a challenge, they learn that it's never as scary as they think. After all, it's *only* anxiety.

## Anxiety is essential for our survival

Avoidance is central to any anxiety disorder because anxiety fills you with an overarching feeling of dread. Dread that something frightening and horrible is about to happen. It makes sense that if there's a potential danger, avoiding it is a perfectly reasonable solution.

With anxiety, avoidance is an evolutionary mechanism of protection.[20] Our ancestors had genuine dangers to avoid. Their survival depended on it. The old saying 'survival of the fittest' would be more accurate if it were 'survival of the fittest and the most alert to danger'. No good being fit if you don't see the danger coming your way in the first place. Those who avoided danger lived to reproduce and the most alert of their offspring would live to do the same.

And so humans have evolved to avoid danger and survive. It just so happens that some brains are far more sensitive to danger than others, resulting in an endless search for safety with an ever-present background level of arousal and alert.

Anxious kids detect danger in places and situations other kids don't because anxious brains are hypersensitive to potential threats. They have wonderful brains that work hard to protect them in circumstances where other kids might feel excitement and a sense of opportunity.

## Avoidance perpetuates anxiety

Unfortunately, avoidance perpetuates anxiety and causes an anxious child to miss out on activities they value. Separation anxiety can see kids missing out on a sleepover at a grandparent's house or a friend's slumber party. There's so much that's awesome about those opportunities. Sleepovers, slumber parties and time spent with grandparents are some of the most enjoyable and memorable experiences for kids – and they're the experiences that promote flourishing mental health. Robust findings from positive psychology tell us that strong connections with friends and family are essential for wellbeing and happiness over a lifetime.

## Positive psychology – a new era

In past decades, countless psychologists dedicated their time and energy to reducing people's suffering. Whether or not that suffering came about via a mental illness, trauma, grief or loss, their aim was to help people move to a place where they experienced less pain and distress, or perhaps even none.

If we think about this on a number line, where zero is in the middle and is flanked by negative numbers in one direction and positive numbers in the other, we can liken the pursuit of psychologists as moving people from a place on the number line less than zero to a place closer to zero, or even zero itself. Zero, for a long time, was the ultimate goal – the place where suffering was reduced and life satisfaction would invariably be improved.

Positive psychology changed all that, with Martin Seligman, PhD, and the late, great Christopher Peterson, PhD, at the helm of this area of research. In his 2008 article for *Psychology Today* Chris Peterson explained:

> Positive psychology is the scientific study of what makes life most worth living. It is a call for psychological science and practice to be as concerned with strength as with weakness; as interested in building the best things in life as in repairing the worst; and as concerned with making the lives of normal people fulfilling as with healing pathology.[21]

Peterson notes that the popularity of positive psychology was increasing when he typed the term into a search engine in May 2008 and found over 419 000 hits. We just did the same, with

26

more than 440 million hits. Peterson would be astonished and proud, to be sure.

If we pop back to our number line for a moment, positive psychology is as much about moving people from less than zero to zero and beyond, as it is about helping people move from zero, or any positive place on the number line, to a place on the line more positive than before. Hence the name.

While avoidance solves the problem of anxiety in the short term, it's a stop sign on the road to flourishing mental health. Avoidance exacerbates anxiety over time, becoming part of a perpetual spiral.

The anxious child who's unable to stay at a friend's house is almost certainly going to struggle when it comes to school camp. The older the kids the higher the stakes. Peers start to notice and ask questions, which can lead to embarrassment or ostracism.

## No family is immune

Macquarie University's Professor Ron Rapee explains that behaviours including hesitation, uncertainty and withdrawal are also forms of avoidance. Even ritualised actions such as frequent handwashing, excessively sharing worries and thoughts with a parent, or repeatedly checking doors are locked, as seen in obsessive-compulsive disorder, are types of avoidance. As a specialist in anxiety disorders across the lifespan, Professor Rapee explains that while avoidance behaviours are fairly consistent across anxiety disorders, there are differences in what triggers them.[22]

It would probably surprise you how many people you know are affected by anxiety. No family is immune, it seems. And it seems one person talking openly about anxiety helps others feel comfortable enough to do the same. Displaying vulnerability gives others permission and confidence. When we see ourselves in someone else's story it empowers us in two ways: to share our own story and to offer our empathy. It's our 'me too', as researcher and author of four number one *New York Times* bestsellers Brené Brown puts it.

In her TED Talk 'Listening to Shame', Dr Brown talks about vulnerability. 'The truth is, vulnerability is not weakness. I define vulnerability as emotional risk, exposure and uncertainty. It fuels our daily lives. And I've come to the belief – this is my twelfth year doing this research – that vulnerability is our most accurate measure of courage.' She continues, 'If we're going to find our way back to each other, vulnerability is going to be that path.'

There's no shame in being anxious. No one chooses it. No one wants it. But we need to talk about it. Being vulnerable is the preferred method of coping. One by one, more people are sharing their story. Watch what happens when you share your story about your own, or your child's, anxiety.

---

### Escaping the custard

Sharing his story for the world to hear is Neil Hughes. In his TED Talk he's funny, a bit awkward, noticeably anxious and ever so endearing. He shares a fantastic analogy for managing anxiety – escape the custard.

Have you ever added water to corn starch and then whacked it? It's quite incredible what happens. When you hit the mixture, it hardens under your hand. When you push gently, your hand sinks into the mixture the way you'd expect. It's called non-Newtonian fluid and behaves differently to most fluids. When a force is applied, the mixture hardens. Apparently the same holds true for certain types of custard. In his TED Talk, Hughes likens the struggle with anxiety to walking on custard: difficult and exhausting – and if you stop, you sink deeply. He also shares some great ideas for avoiding custard traps.

---

# 2

# What's causing the epidemic?

Why are so many kids anxious? What changes have caused great numbers of children to struggle with their mental health?

It's easy to point the finger at technology. After all, for something to have such a profound impact on the mental health of children, it's important to explore a link between this change and the culture in which they're living. On the timeline of human history sits an Apple (with one leaf and a bite out of one side) marking the time where the internet, or World Wide Web as it was called, became readily accessible.

Life was forever changed.

The causes underlying the epidemic of anxiety among children and teenagers are many and varied. Some are unchangeable or unavoidable, including: genetic factors,[1] early trauma, stressful life experiences including bullying[2] or the death of a loved one, parental mental health,[3] world events[4] and natural disasters.[5]

Other contributors are within the realm of parental influence. Let's explore that now.

## What have screens got to do with it?

> *It's not an exaggeration to describe iGen as being on the brink of the worst mental-health crisis in decades.*
>
> — Jean Twenge, 2017

As a generational researcher Professor Jean Twenge has never seen such stark changes in mental health as she has for the generation of kids, teens and young adults born between 1995 and 2012. She attributes these changes to the use of phones.

'They grew up with cell phones, had an Instagram page before they started high school, and do not remember a time before the Internet,' writes Twenge in her popular book *iGen*.[6] It was in 2012 that the fast-growing number of Americans owning a smartphone tipped 50 per cent. Smartphone ownership was skyrocketing in Australia at the same time.

In 2012 the Australian Communications and Media Authority reported that over 8.67 million Australian adults owned a smart-phone, up 104 per cent from the previous year.[7]

The number of smartphones owned by Australians has continued to grow. By now, the market for smartphones is just about saturated.

## Time on devices – a double-edged sword

With devices in their hands, apps and the internet at their disposal and/or social media and video games connecting them with their friends, there are two distinct ways in which screen time impacts on kids' mental health. First, content accessed via screens may be upsetting, frightening or confusing. Second, there's an opportunity cost in terms of the activities that kids avoid such as physical activity, meeting with friends and spending time outdoors that have a positive impact on mental health and wellbeing, especially anxiety.

When kids spend time on devices, including phones, tablets and video games, they're not playing with or spending time with their friends, nor are they moving around, reading, playing sport, using their imaginations, getting bored, nurturing their creativity, doing their homework, interacting with their family or sleeping.

These activities and many more contribute to flourishing mental health. Every hour on a device is one less hour kids have to develop healthy lifestyle habits and develop positive views of themselves by cultivating their character and exploring their values. Other activities that fall by the wayside include having fun and connecting with their brothers or sisters and parents, learning, thinking, exploring, building on their relationships, risk-taking and contributing to their communities.

The more time children and adolescents spend on screens the lower their psychological wellbeing.[8] Every hour a child is on a device is an hour they're not developing the skills, strategies and resources to protect and bolster their mental health.

Excessive screen time puts kids' psychological and physical health at risk. More screen time equates to less movement and is predictably related to increased obesity.[9] Obesity elevates the chances of children experiencing problems with their heart health, metabolic health and blood sugar regulation. Obese children are also more likely to be bullied, which contributes to, or exacerbates, anxiety.

## Sword edge one – time on devices

### How screen time affects sleep

How do you feel when you wake without having enough sleep? You have that sluggish, tired feeling that makes it hard to get moving and leaves you feeling irritable! We know intuitively how sleep affects our moods. As adults, we know how it impacts on our kids too.

Sleep is essential for good mental health. Kids need more sleep than adults.

Irrespective of the viewed content that may make it hard for a child to fall asleep after using a screen, exposure to the light emitted from a screen at night also interferes with sleep. This is because light is what enables all of us to keep our body clock ticking along in time with our environment.

## The blue light sleep bandit

Screens emit a blue, short-wavelength light that interferes with our natural circadian rhythm. It impacts on the production of the sleep hormone melatonin, also known as the 'hormone of darkness', more so than light of longer wavelengths.

Levels of melatonin rise and fall over twenty-four hours and help regulate the sleep–wake cycle. Melatonin rises in the two hours before sleep, bringing with it a drowsy, 'I'm ready for bed' feeling; and peaks in the early hours of the morning, around 3 or 4 a.m. When melatonin production is suppressed by the blue light emitted from screens, it impacts on the ability to fall asleep as well as the quality of sleep during the night.[10]

The body clock is regulated by light exposure, so when screens delay sleep onset and reduce total sleep time routinely, it has long-term effects on sleep and wake cycles, and ultimately on mental health.

## How is it different for adolescents?

The impact of blue light from devices at night is confounded by the naturally occurring delay in melatonin release for adolescents. In her article for *The Conversation*, senior research fellow from the University of Minnesota Kyla Wahlstrom advocates later starting times for high school students, owing to the biology of the teenage brain. Wahlstrom explains:

For virtually all adolescents, the secretion of melatonin doesn't begin until about 10.45 p.m. and continues until about 8 a.m. This means that most teenagers are unable to fall asleep until melatonin secretion begins. It's hard to wake up until the melatonin secretion stops. This fixed pattern of melatonin secretion in teens changes back to an individual's genetically preferred sleep/wake timing once puberty is over.[11]

Melatonin is also important for mental health as it helps regulate anxiety, which is another reason to support anxious children to develop regular sleep patterns.[12]

## Sunlight, serotonin and sleep

Residual melatonin upon waking is quickly broken down when the curtains are opened, exposing the eyes to sunlight. This also helps melatonin production to occur sooner that same evening, making it easier to fall asleep. Although they might object, the sooner sunlight is streaming into the bedroom of an anxious child in the morning, the better they will be.

Serotonin, known as a 'feel-good chemical' in the brain, is produced during daylight hours. It plays an important role in the regulation of emotions and behaviour. Another reason to open up those curtains first thing! Exposure to natural sunlight enhances serotonin production,[13] and optimum levels of serotonin result in more positive moods and a calm, yet focused, mental outlook.[14]

It's likely you've experienced the effects of low serotonin. Can you relate to the parent who says that 'the happy, relaxed and playful mum clocks off at 8 p.m. and that's when grumpy mum takes over'? It's in kids' best interests to go to bed before the change of shift!

As the day wears on and melatonin begins to rise, serotonin in the brain is falling. If the demands of the day are still high on parents in the late afternoon, the reduction in serotonin can lead to grumpiness, irritability, impatience, fatigue, an inability to focus and even anger.[15] Interestingly, nutritional biochemist Dr Judith Wurtman, author of *The Serotonin Power Diet*, explains that eating around 30 grams of sugar or starchy carbohydrate with a couple of grams of healthy fats and a few grams of protein will produce serotonin within half an hour, bringing with it positive changes in mood. Bring on the (healthy) snacks!

Serotonin is important for regulating anxiety. A group of medications that are prescribed to treat anxiety are called selective serotonin reuptake inhibitors, or SSRIs.[16] They work by increasing the level of serotonin in the brain, but not by artificially elevating serotonin. Instead, they make more serotonin available by blocking the reuptake (reabsorption).

## Tired and emotional – the role of the amygdala

When we're tired, we're more likely to pay attention to negative events and influences than we would if we're well rested.

The amygdala (which we'll explore in more depth in Chapter 3) is the emotional regulation centre of the brain. One research study compared activity in the amygdala in response to unpleasant images in adults who hadn't slept for thirty-five hours, with adults who had enjoyed ample sleep. The amygdala showed increased activity in both groups when unpleasant images were shown, but in the group of people who were tired from lack of sleep the activation in the amygdala was remarkably 60 per cent higher.[17]

This means the amygdala is hypersensitive to negative events and stimuli when we're tired. Since anxious kids already have an amygdala that is hypersensitive to threat, by ensuring they're getting plenty of sleep the added influence of hypersensitivity due to tiredness is lessened or removed.

The same research group also found that lack of sleep interfered with the ability of the prefrontal cortex to regulate the amygdala's function. The prefrontal cortex is the front third of the brain, located behind the eyes and forehead. It's the brain region responsible for complex thinking, problem-solving, decision-making and emotional regulation. We'll delve deeper into the role of the prefrontal cortex in Chapter 3.

## Potential risks of social media

### Wired for comparison

*Comparison is the thief of joy.*

— Theodore Roosevelt

From a biological point of view, humans are wired to compare themselves with others.

In the days of early humans, safety in numbers was a big driver of comparison. Those who were constantly comparing their efforts to other members of their society were better able to ensure that they were meeting the expectations of the group. Being considered a valuable member of the group greatly reduced the risk of being abandoned. This risk to safety naturally meant that not measuring up was a signal to the amygdala of danger. We know that the amygdala's role in protecting us from danger is what underlies anxiety. Those who were wired to compare survived, their genes passing on to subsequent generations.

The internet now makes it easy to compare yourself to others. Want a dose of 'wish we were drinking cocktails by the pool on a tropical island during the summer holidays'? If so, open up your Facebook or Instagram feed and you can compare the day away in the comfort of your own home.

Without realising it, when young people view social media they're constantly making comparisons. What they often overlook is that they're measuring their own real life against everyone else's highlights reel.

## FOMO, aka fear of missing out

Before the internet, kids learned they'd missed out on an invitation to a party either in the lead-up to the event or in the days following, if at all. Perhaps a lunchtime rumour or an unthinking comment by a friend would let the cat out of the bag. Now everyone knows because pictures from a party are posted on social media before many kids have finished their first handful of chips.

This type of exclusion again plays into the brain's propensity for comparison, which leaves many young people feeling excluded and isolated.

While it's natural, and sensible, to encourage young people to minimise their time on social media, it's quite difficult for them. Smartphones and apps are deliberately designed to be addictive and keep us scrolling.

Unlike ads on TV which interrupt viewing, or the end of a TV program which does the same, there are no 'stopping' cues on social media platforms. It's a never-ending stream of stimulation and pseudo connection. FOMO not only relates to missing out on social invitations, it also drives young people to keep scrolling so they don't miss something 'important'.

As they scroll they experience the drip, drip, drip of dopamine, a reward chemical in the brain that feels good and fuels more scrolling,[18] compelling kids to spend hours on devices.

## Always connected but never more lonely

We've all heard that it takes a village to raise kids but we usually look at this from the point of view of having many pairs of hands to step in and help when needed. The real reason it takes a village is because in a village there are lots of kids. A child has many friends to play with, to learn from, to build relationship skills with, to talk to, to solve problems with, to climb trees with, to create games with and to have fun with.

Relationships are at the core of human happiness, for all of us.

Screens have interrupted kids' relationships in ways that could have long-term consequences for their mental health. Evidence suggests that they're constantly connected with each other through technology, but they've never been so lonely.[19] Ironically, kids with phones don't use them to make phone calls. They message and communicate via their keyboards, often for hours at a time.

Non-profit organisation Common Sense Media undertook a census so they could gain a better understanding of media use by tweens (8–12-year-olds) and teens (13–18-year-olds). They made astonishing findings. Tweens were found to spend an average of 4.5 hours per day on screen media for entertainment, while teenagers averaged 6.5 hours of screen media per day. This doesn't include time spent using media for school or homework.[20] In general, girls tend to spend more time connecting with each other via social media, whereas boys spend more time gaming.

Connecting via social media can strengthen relationships, but it's face-to-face interaction where kids and teens connect on a deeper level. Through these types of interactions kids are able to learn from the nuances of facial expression and another person's tone of voice and body language, and avoid the pitfalls of misinterpreting emojis and written text.

## Other screen factors that could be playing a role in anxiety

Communicating and posting via screens involves anticipation and disappointment. Text messages don't convey emotion the way a personal conversation will. Even the use of emojis, which are prolific, are hard to interpret at times.

Waiting for a reply to a text causes stress for some young people. While they're waiting they're anything but mindful. Their thoughts are often centred on checking and rechecking their devices so they can read any reply as soon as it lands. On the flip side, teens will deliberately put off replying if they want to make a friend or partner sweat for a while.

The use of social media impacts young people's everyday thinking. If we could amplify some of their thoughts on any given day we'd hear them asking questions like:

Why isn't everyone 'liking' my picture?
How does she manage to look perfect in every photograph?
Why hasn't he responded yet?
Is she annoyed at me? I can't tell from this text.
Why hasn't he followed me back?
Why is everyone else having more fun than I am?
Is that an 'all good' smiley face or does it mean something else?

## The need to be liked

The need to be 'liked' both in an online and offline world is strong for young people. Teenage girls especially will remove photos from their social media feeds if they don't get enough 'likes'.

Not getting enough 'likes' impacts sense of self for some, potentially contributing to anxiety. Being on the receiving end of outright negativity such as cyberbullying has even more potential to negatively impact a young person's mental health.

In the days before screens, a young person who was being bullied at school could at least escape it outside of school. That's no longer the case for young people who use social media. There isn't an escape from what the brain considers a threat, and so there are links between bullying or cyberbullying and anxiety.[21]

Cyberbullying is bullying online. It encompasses being hurt by someone using technology via email, chat rooms, text messages, discussion groups, social media, instant messaging or websites.[22] In one study, 68 per cent of young people who had experienced cyberbullying had received a nasty private message; 41 per cent had rumours posted about them online.[23] In the case of cyber-bullying, the ill-treatment of a child is witnessed by many more people than when it happens in person, amplifying the humiliation. In addition, a bully often hides behind a false username, making their behaviour hard to track and stop.

## Sword edge two – time away from other activities

Screen time is alluring. Many parents experience difficulties helping their young people to manage screen time to ensure they're living rich, full and well-rounded lives. As we mentioned earlier, screens contribute to anxiety in many different ways, but we can't overlook the activities that children and young people are missing when they're online.

Each new day is a chance for parents to create opportunities for their kids to participate in activities that boost their mental health and build their resilience to mental illness. Here are some examples:

- spending time together as a family
- hanging out with friends
- playing sport
- playing at the park
- beach fun
- drawing
- reading
- bike riding
- baking
- volunteering
- training for sport
- helping out around the home
- working part-time
- visiting family
- playing with pets
- walking to the local shops.

Screen time doesn't have to be abandoned for children who are experiencing anxiety. It's all about moderation. If children are engaging in a variety of activities in addition to their screen time, it's less likely to be harmful to their mental health and more likely to have a positive influence on their lives.

## Finally, some good news

It's not all doom and gloom. As part of a healthy and balanced lifestyle there's good that comes from spending time on devices when young people are savvy about privacy and smart about their digital use.

There are many benefits for young people when they connect with friends via social networking sites including Instagram, Snapchat, Facebook and gaming sites. The online world is a place for young people to 'hang out' with their friends after school and on weekends. Used wisely, it serves to strengthen their identity and friendships at the same time.

Young people have a great time together online by sending funny memes, making videos or using amusing filters on their selfies, to name a few. They build their social skills through text-based banter, exchanges on social apps and comments left on social media posts. Social media also offers an opportunity for a young person who feels isolated and lonely to connect with and feel part of a community or group, bolstering their self-esteem and mental health.

The internet and social media also presents opportunities for young people to better understand and take action on community or global issues that they have an interest in, such as climate change or an accumulation of plastic waste on their local beach.

The internet is a great resource for a young person who is experiencing anxiety and wants to understand more about it. It's a confidential and anonymous place where answers to questions, at websites of reputable mental health providers such as Beyond Blue and ReachOut, are easily found. There are support services online, trusted sources of information and useful programs, such as The Brave Program, moodgym and our Parenting Anxious Kids course.[24]

## Busy lives, stressed parents

Decades ago it was envisaged that technology would add hours of leisure time to every week. In 1965 IBM economist Joseph Froomkin predicted that automation would lead to a twenty-hour work week 'creating a mass leisure class'.[25] We're still waiting.

Despite the predictions, technology continues to underpin a working culture where parents are constantly connected to work via the modern-day version of the bat phone. It's rare for working parents to clock on and clock off, leaving unfinished business, unanswered emails and loose ends for the next 'shift'. Technological advancements are further eating up precious leisure time as employees and employers alike are constantly 'on call' in the 'new' 24-hour economy. This adds to the busyness of already very full days.

Australia ranked twenty-seventh out of thirty-seven countries when it comes to work–life balance in a 2017 report by the Organisation for Economic Co-operation and Development.[26] Countries including the Russian Federation, Czech Republic and Slovenia fare better than Australia when it comes to annual number of hours worked each year, and paid leave, including holiday, maternity and paternity leave. Tipping-points have been identified at which working more hours impacts the mental health of men (43.5 hours per week) and women (thirty-nine hours per week).[27] The differences are attributed to men working more paid hours and doing less in the home. Raising kids who flourish is challenging enough without the added struggle of managing your own mental health.

Other Australian research reveals that when parents are struggling to balance long working hours and work responsibilities with family life it negatively impacts children's mental health.[28] On the upside, when balance is regained, children's mental health improves too.

## Declining 'mental bandwidth'

Parents are busier than ever before, with long working hours, extracurricular activities to get kids to, and endless household chores. Add to the mix the need to catch up with their own friends, answer text messages, spend time with the kids and fit in activities that boost their own health and wellbeing, it's no wonder parents feel they just don't have the 'mental bandwidth' to cope with much more at times. A heavy mental load feels stressful and stress is equally as contagious as anxiety.

Stressed parents are less likely to interact with their children with warmth, affection and sensitivity. They're also more likely to overreact and use more controlling techniques when it comes to managing behaviour than parents who are less stressed.[29]

## Stay-at-home parents can struggle too

Even for parents who don't work outside of the home, family life is often hectic and rushed. The constant trips between home and kinder for three- and four-year-olds mean many parents with preschool-age children feel they just about live in their cars. When children are at school the hours between drop-off and pick-up seem to fly by too. Parents can feel as though their own needs aren't being met and time spent together as a family, or individually with children, can be relegated because parents become depleted in both time and energy.

## Is busy a badge of honour?

We challenge you to ask an adult today how they're doing and not hear them say 'busy'. It's almost as though if we're not busy, we're not worthy.

Take a moment to think of how much you hustle each day. Are you sitting down to eat breakfast or taking a proper break in the middle of your workday for lunch? Do you tap away at the keyboard while you're on the phone at work, or grab the duster or hang out the washing so you're not spending idle time chatting if you're at home? Do you try to get those last few tasks done before you leave for work or school drop-off in the morning because there's so much to do when you return home? Do you multi-task in the kitchen each evening? Perhaps you listen to some reading homework, help with maths questions or try to catch up on the day's events while being careful not to peel your finger along with the carrots? Do you walk fast? Do you drop off your kids at their sport only to dash to the supermarket to pick up some staples? Do you stop? Ever?

Our guess is not often.

When you're stressed and depleted, it's harder to be present and available for your kids.

If you're having a tough day, are worried or feel badly about a particular incident that's happened, you won't launch into a conversation about it with your partner or a friend if you know they're rushed. Intuitively you understand it's better to wait until a more appropriate time to open up and share what you're thinking and feeling.

Kids are the same. They'll wait for a time when they feel comfortable and connected enough to share what's going on for them. This explains why many meaningful conversations happen at bedtime.

## Doing too much for them

Parents tend to do more for their kids than is needed when they find themselves pressed for time. It's faster and easier to do tasks for kids than allow them time to work through them on their own. But that doesn't teach them new skills, or responsibility for themselves or for their mishaps.

We'll use an example we've both experienced as parents. The kids knock a 2-litre bottle of milk off the bench onto the floor while making breakfast. It just about floods the kitchen. But they clean it up and by the time they let you know what happened, only the faint swirls of drying milk on the floor remain. You need to mop the floor but the bulk of the clean-up has been done. No one gets upset and you're able to move on with getting ready for school.

We recommend that you view your role as a guide or coach for your child. You will need to be patient enough to allow your child to learn from their own mistakes and be prepared to repeat some earlier lessons without becoming frustrated or annoyed.

It's easy to overreact when you're a busy parent. Stressed parents generally don't have the bandwidth to respond thoughtfully and manage problems well. If stress and upset becomes your default setting when your kids make mistakes, it will eventually become a default setting for them too.

Once something's broken, it's broken. Once something's spilled, it's spilled. It can't be undone. Taking responsibility by framing a mistake as an opportunity to learn is the most helpful response you can make.

## Overscheduled kids

There's a general consensus that today's kids are overscheduled. Some kids are so busy that they're doing their homework in the car. We are aware that some families have extracurricular activities scheduled for their children almost every day of the week.

The busyness of life for kids has a twofold impact on their mental health and wellbeing. They feel rushed much of the time if their schedules are full. While structured activities can foster good mental health via the exercise, time in nature and friendships they promote, an inordinate amount of time spent at scheduled activities is time children are not involved in other healthy activities that bolster their mental wellbeing. Playing outside, hanging out with friends, riding bikes, making up games, spending time in the sunshine at the park or in the garden, climbing trees, building or having enough spare time to feel bored are all activities which nurture mental health.

The time children have for free play, defined as playing alone or with other kids without any adult input, has sharply declined over the past fifty years. In his article published in the *American Journal of Play*, Peter Gray, PhD, a psychology research professor at Boston College, links the decline in play with the rise in anxiety, depression, feelings of helplessness and suicide in children.[30] He explains that play promotes positive mental health by enabling children to develop interests and competence, learn how to make decisions, solve problems, follow rules, exert self-control, learn how to regulate their emotions, make friends, get along with others as equals and experience joy.

## Avoid the news

Kids who are anxious often feel threatened when they hear events happening in the media. The news is almost all 'bad' news. Younger children struggle to understand that a world event is likely a world away from them. They may hear on the news, particularly on TV or the radio, that there's a war in the Middle East and experience the threat of danger as if it were on their doorstep.

Children and young people who experience anxiety are often plagued with uncontrollable and irrational thoughts and worry. Exposing them to the events of the day via the news, whether close to home or far away, has the potential to fuel anxious thoughts and feelings. In these instances, the news is best avoided wherever possible. If it's unavoidable then explain any news they are exposed to in age-appropriate ways.

# Part 2

# Understanding anxiety

Children have a natural tendency to ask questions. They're curious by nature, wanting to know how the world works. Adults around them generally supply the information they need to get by. Anxiety is no different. Though they may not think to ask, educating them about their anxiety is laying the foundations upon which they will build their understanding and management. This process is called psychoeducation.

In this section of the book we'll introduce you to the various 'players' in an anxious brain and the roles they perform. You'll learn exactly what anxiety is, what's happening in the brain, how it shows up, common types of anxiety and more.

The symptoms of anxiety become more evident over time, gradually impacting on a child's thinking, how they're feeling and their behaviour. Displaying symptoms of anxiety doesn't necessarily mean an anxiety disorder is at play. By keeping an eye on changes and keeping a journal of what you observe, you'll be well placed if the time comes for you to seek professional help.

That said, we strongly recommend you visit your general practitioner if you suspect, even slightly, that your child is struggling with anxiety. We know of many families who have done this only to be reassured that what their child is experiencing is no cause for concern, that it falls within normal developmental ranges and that it should settle of its own accord. In the event that an anxiety disorder is suspected, seeking professional support means you have put the ball in motion to help them with their anxiety. The sooner they start the better.

# 3

# Anxiety explained

## What is anxiety?

When any of us have reason to worry, feel pressure or feel stressed about a situation or an upcoming event or challenge, we can experience anxiety. As you now know, in these cases the anxiety settles down when the stressful event, challenge or circumstances pass. This is a completely normal human response to a stressor and is temporary. When a person has an anxiety disorder, these feelings don't go away.

Children and teenagers experience anxiety for any number of reasons. Even if you're not entirely sure where your child's anxiety comes from, the explanation of what's happening in the brain is the same. At the heart of anxiety is a brain that works hard to protect a child. This helps explain why anxious children and teenagers, like anxious adults, often experience persistent, excessive and unrealistic worry, fears and even a sense of dread. Their brain is overly sensitive to potential threat, influencing their thoughts as well as how they feel and act.

The brains of anxious children are on high alert. They experience symptoms of their anxiety as a result of events, thoughts or circumstances where there is a clear cause and effect. At other times, anxiety comes unbidden, with no apparent cause or reason to help understand its origin. This is often baffling for children and parents but is common.

Anxious thoughts and feelings are often out of proportion to the triggering event. Anxious thoughts are frequently irrational and may seem ridiculous to parents. At times children and teens recognise that their thinking is irrational, but can't help it or how it makes them feel.

As a parent you don't necessarily need to understand why your newborn baby is crying to respond in helpful and loving ways. The same holds true when responding to anxiety. You can respond in the same way whether you know where the anxiety is coming from or not.

## Sam's story

Sam was being bullied at school. He was in Year Nine when he was diagnosed with anxiety after enduring bullying on and off by the same boy since starting high school. Sam had tried everything. He'd talked to his parents and his teachers. He had tried to ignore the bully. He had taken himself off all of his social media accounts to avoid more taunting outside of school hours, but still the bully persisted.

Sam would often be cornered by the bully and taunted while the bully's friends watched and laughed.

Sam's anxiety started out as difficulty breathing every now and again, but over time his symptoms progressed to multiple daily worries, tears, anger and panic attacks.

There came a time when Sam found it extremely difficult to even get out of bed. He described feeling as though he was having a heart attack, with pain and a heaviness in his chest and dizzy feelings that stopped him from being able to get up and function.

Anxiety is the body's response to fear. Sam feared his bully for good reason, and it caused him anxiety that eventually progressed to an anxiety disorder. An anxiety disorder is diagnosed when anxiety gets in the way of day-to-day functioning and enjoyment of life.

What's important to remember is that the anxiety response in the brain and the body is the same whether the fear is in response to a known threat or one that is only perceived or imagined. Once the body's alarm system has been set off, the cascade of events that define anxiety are the same.

## Can you relate?

If you're finding it hard to relate to the experience of your anxious child, you're not alone. Parents who don't have an anxiety disorder may find it difficult to tap into what it feels like, potentially standing in the way of their ability to genuinely empathise with their anxious child.

As parents, we know you want nothing more than to show your child that you get it, and to show them that you relate to how they're feeling. To that end, we want to take a moment to ask you a question: Have you ever lost one of your children? Even momentarily?

Surprisingly, almost every hand goes up when we ask this question in our presentations. Most of us, at one time or another, have had the terrifying experience of temporarily losing one of our kids. Be it for a minute in the supermarket or twenty minutes in a crowd, parents describe feeling a hot rush of blood through their body, a sinking stomach and thoughts of awful reasons why their child might have vanished. Every sense is on high alert and there's an overwhelming urge to locate the missing child as quickly as possible. Even when the child has been found, those feelings hang around for a while.

Anxiety triggers the release of neurochemicals, and those chemicals swirl around the body long after parent and child have been reunited, or any other stressor has passed.

Even if you're lucky enough never to have 'misplaced' a child, try tapping into how you have felt before a big exam or a job interview. It will help you to connect more with how your anxious child is feeling.

## Not broken, no way

A common theme among anxious kids is that there's something wrong with them. That they're somehow broken. Let us tell you right now they're not. Not even a bit. Anxious children simply have a brain that is almost always on high alert for potential threats. Their brains work overtime to protect them from danger.

Explaining to anxious children that there's a name for what they're experiencing, and that there are likely two or three other kids in their classroom who also have an amazing and protective brain like theirs, helps them to understand that they're not alone. When kids learn that their experience isn't unique, that in fact there are millions of other kids all over the world dealing with anxiety, and that, importantly, it's manageable, they will feel reassured.

They're not broken. They're amazing. Most kids who experience anxiety are thoughtful, sensitive, caring, loving, kind, generous, funny and compassionate; and so loved. Let them know they're enough just as they are and that any help they need is akin to learning a new skill to manage their brain's alarm system. They don't need fixing; they need understanding, love, empathy, support and sometimes professional help.

## The body's alarm system

Anxiety is the body's way of protecting us when we're in danger or when there is danger around the corner. It's an age-old system within the brain, rooted in our biology.

It's completely normal to feel anxious from time to time. A child might feel anxious about speaking in front of their class or competing in the sport they love. A teenager might feel anxious about an interview for a part-time job, asking someone out on a date or a test at school.

As well as improving memory and increasing alertness, short-term stress and the anxious feelings that follow act as a motivator to do more revision or be better prepared.

We can liken our anxiety response to a smoke alarm. The alarm is designed to alert us to fire, a danger that poses a threat to our life. When there's a house fire, the smoke alarm sounds. It does its job, letting everyone in the home know of the danger so they act to stay safe.

In a similar way, our anxiety response is a protective system, designed to protect us from life-threatening danger. If our fight-or-flight system simply got us activated to escape real danger, the way a smoke detector goes off in a house fire, no problem.

Anxiety becomes a problem when the mind's alarm system is extremely sensitive and responds when there's no genuine danger present. It's as if the body's alarm system sounds in response to the equivalent of burned toast.

Kids with anxiety often experience the symptoms when they're quite safe; the danger is only imagined.

## Meet the players

### The amygdala

Anxiety is linked to abnormal functioning of the amygdala, an almond-shaped region of the brain that receives input from our senses – typically our senses of sight and hearing. The amygdala plays a key role in the processing of emotions too, which is why anxiety is often accompanied by big emotions such as sadness and anger.

As we have already touched upon, brain scans of anxious people show more activity in the amygdala than in people without anxiety.[1] The amygdala has also been found to be larger in anxious children,[2] and given it is known as the 'fear centre' of the brain, it makes sense that an anxious brain with a bigger amygdala has a bigger response to danger, real or not.

In essence, when the amygdala senses danger it sends a distress signal to prepare the body for action to face the danger or flee. This is activated by the sympathetic nervous system and is known as the fight-or-flight response.

## The fight-or-flight response

The fight-or-flight response is an instinctive life-saving response to danger. It's not meant to be constantly activated the way it often is for anxious kids. This is one of the reasons anxiety feels so exhausting.

The 'fight' part of this response helps explain the anger and aggressive behaviour displayed by some anxious children and teenagers. The 'flight' part of the response helps explain the avoidance that is so common with anxiety. There are also times when kids just freeze, neither fighting nor fleeing. They're just too anxious to do anything.

The fight-or-flight response prepares the body in a variety of ways to stand up and fight the danger or flee. It triggers the release of adrenaline and hormones that result in physical changes including increased heart rate and increased breathing rate that 'power up' the body for conflict or escape.

All these changes show up suddenly, and leave a person feeling anything from unpleasant to awful. The feelings make kids and teens feel distressed and they want them to stop as soon as possible.

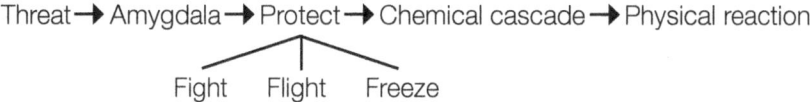

**Figure 1:** The fight-or-flight response

## The prefrontal cortex – no time for thinking

When faced with danger, the amygdala signals the body to fight or flee without the need to think first. It happens almost instantaneously. The amygdala senses danger and signals the cascade of events for fight or flight to happen without input from the decision-making part of the brain, the prefrontal cortex.

If the amygdala is the watchdog in the yard, and the fight-or-flight response is the dog attacking or escaping, the prefrontal cortex is the cat sitting high on the fence watching the show. The watchdog attacks or escapes knowing there's no time to ask the cat for more information about what's going on. In anxious kids, the watchdog is (almost) always jumping at shadows.

Put simply, anxiety short-circuits the decision-making process and for good reason.[3] When it comes to life or death, 'act first think later' is faster. In *The Whole-Brain Child*, Daniel Siegel, a Harvard graduate and seasoned clinical professor of psychiatry, explains how it was his amygdala that prompted him to scream 'stop' when he saw a rattlesnake on the path ahead of where he was hiking with his son, even before he consciously knew what was happening.

He writes an amusing account of the process that would have occurred had his prefrontal cortex been included in the reaction: 'Oh no! There's a snake up ahead of my son. Now would be a good time to warn him. I wish I had warned him a couple of seconds ago, rather than going through this series of cogitations that led me to the decision to warn him.'

It makes sense that this part of the brain is left out of the loop.

As well as being responsible for decision-making, the pre-frontal cortex is involved in:

- planning
- behaviour in social settings
- imagination
- judgement
- verbal reasoning
- problem-solving
- sustained attention
- the ability to deal with novelty
- the ability to differentiate between conflicting thoughts
- consequences
- working towards a goal
- the ability to suppress urges that could be deemed socially unacceptable.

Perhaps when reading this list you're making connections between the behaviour of your anxious child and why they might be struggling with one or some of the skills and behaviours that need input from the prefrontal cortex.

Anxiety impacts on children in ways that can be better understood when parents pay attention to what their child thinks, how they feel and what they do. Sometimes you'll see these referred to as cognition, physiology and behaviour. No matter what you call it, it makes much more sense when you keep in mind what's happening in the brain and body.

## What happens to thinking in an anxious brain?

When children and teens are feeling anxious, their amygdala has sensed danger and triggered their fight-or-flight response. It can happen anywhere: in a classroom before a quiz, while they're in their room reading a book, watching the news, walking to school, playing a game, shooting hoops or texting with a friend.

Worry is a common feature of anxiety. It's a helpful way to protect us from danger because we worry about what threatens us. Have you had a skin check? Perhaps you've done so after noticing a skin spot that worried you. Your worry may have indeed saved your life. However, worry that's frequent, excessive, unfounded and irrational impacts quality of life.

It happens when something is viewed by the amygdala as a threat. The worry starts and continues because the mind knows that constant focus on the threat may just be the trick to averting serious danger. A worrying mind reflects on events of the past, or fast-forwards to a possible future. Helping anxious kids remain more mindful, with their attention in the present, brings them such relief.

With practice, mindfulness helps worrying thoughts become less 'sticky' – it becomes easier to detach from them and get on with living life. Mindfulness decreases the size and reactivity of the amygdala, increases connectivity between the amygdala and the prefrontal cortex and increases the density and activity of the calming prefrontal cortex.[4]

## Bad thoughts

We all have tens of thousands of thoughts each day. There's no consensus among scientists precisely how many but we know, as adults, we're easily able to dismiss most of our thoughts without realising we're doing so. If we do notice 'bad thoughts' we're usually able to move on and forget about them, knowing they're meaningless. It happens almost instantaneously.

Some children can judge many of their thoughts as 'bad'. They can have thoughts that they recognise as being unkind, unfair, hurtful, untrue, mean, sexual in nature or even harmful. These thoughts are distressing for anxious kids. They don't want the thoughts. They don't understand where they're coming from and they think badly of themselves for having them. A child experiencing intrusive thoughts that they can't dismiss might be experiencing obsessions.

It's common for kids with obsessive thoughts to regularly confess whatever they're thinking, typically to one of their parents. They do this to get the reassurance they need that their thoughts are untrue and they're not a bad person. This can become a compulsion. They need to share their thoughts to relieve their anxiety. Other compulsions can include handwashing, counting, tapping or pulling at their hair. A child with these experiences might be diagnosed with obsessive-compulsive disorder.

## They need the help from your prefrontal cortex

As their parent you will usually know when your child's thinking is left of centre, irrational or disproportionate to the circumstances. You have a good sense of when their thoughts are trivial and when there's no danger, just like the cat sitting on the fence sees that the watchdog is jumping at shadows. But your child can't see their situation from the same perspective. If you attempt to appeal to the part of their brain responsible for problem-solving, decision-making and verbal reasoning, you're not likely to get far because in effect, that part of their brain, their prefrontal cortex, has gone offline. It will come back online eventually. For this reason we recommend that you save conversations about the circumstances that brought on their anxiety for well after the event when their brains are ready to take in information.

Now that you understand the role of the prefrontal cortex you can see how anxiety impacts a child's thinking. You can see how access is denied to that part of the brain when kids are anxious.

Working with children to manage their anxiety is more effective when done in between anxious moments. When they're feeling calm and relaxed you'll be better able to help them develop their understanding of what's happening in their brain and cultivate approaches that enable them to manage their anxiety such as helpful thinking skills, and breathing and mind-fulness exercises.

This is why anxiety impacts learning for many kids. When children are anxious their brain is working hard to keep them safe; memory and learning are then affected. The anxiety makes it hard for kids not only to think, but to concentrate for any length of time. Their brain is in survival mode while the prefrontal cortex is offline. Helping them transfer their anxiety management strategies to the classroom is vital, as is involving their teacher to support their efforts.

## How does anxiety impact physiology?

In addition to impacting thinking, anxiety causes a range of physical changes in the body. Part of the fight-or-flight response is the surge of neurochemicals, including adrenaline, that power up the body to deal with the 'dangerous' situation at hand.

When considered from the point of view of preparing the body for fight or flight, the physiological changes accompanying anxiety make sense.

• The heart beats faster to pump more blood around the body, providing oxygen as a fuel for muscles and other vital organs.
• The breathing rate increases to bring more oxygen to the bloodstream.
• Small airways in the lungs open up, enabling more oxygen to be taken in with each breath.
• Blood is shunted from the digestive system to the limbs.
• The body's cooling system ramps up in the expectation of movement, making the skin feel clammy or sweaty.
• Extra oxygen is sent to the brain to increase alertness.
• Vision, hearing and other senses become sharper.
• Blood sugars and fats are released from temporary storage in the body to provide energy.[5]

Initial changes happen almost immediately and once the release of adrenaline begins to slow down, cortisol, a stress hormone, is released to keep the body powered up if the brain continues to sense danger.

It's no wonder anxiety feels the way it does. The body is primed in every way possible to fight for life or flee to safety, and yet nothing happens. None of these changes are put to use because an anxious child doesn't have a life-threatening situation on their hands. They don't need to move a muscle. They are all powered up with nowhere to go.

For this reason anxious kids can feel shaky, flushed, fired up, uncertain, threatened, reactive, impatient and like they don't know what to do with themselves or are unable to sit still. They can feel nauseous or vomit because blood has been shunted away from their stomach to their arms and legs where it's needed most.

This happens quickly as the sympathetic nervous system takes over the running of the 'show'. Anxious kids need their para-sympathetic nervous system, the 'rest-and-digest' system, to take over. The only conscious control we have over the activity of this system is through breathing. We'll talk more about that in Chapter 10.

## Why is behaviour affected by anxiety?

Anxious kids can be quiet, shy, agreeable, sensitive and empa-thetic; they can be perfectionists and deep thinkers. They can also be disruptive, irritable, easily upset, angry and oppositional. When children are regularly in fight-or-flight mode it's perfectly understandable that some will withdraw and shy away from any perceived danger or threat, while others will face up to the threat, often overwhelmed by a distressing urge to confront whatever it is that sets off their amygdala.

When anxiety results in changes in behaviour it's often mis-interpreted. The behaviour of an anxious child at school can be very different to their behaviour at home where they feel safe and relatively relaxed. Anxious kids who 'fight' rather than 'flee' can be thought of as troublemaking, defiant, inattentive, disruptive, intimidating and even a danger to others.

## Shani's story

Shani was in Grade Five at an all-girls private school. She'd always loved school. She was well-liked by her teacher, had lovely friends and loved learning. Over recent months her efforts in class and the quality of her schoolwork had declined. She made up excuses to stay home from school and when she did go, she struggled to concentrate and get her work done.

Her mum was contacted by the school after a teacher noticed offensive drawings in Shani's diary. They were of her older sister. Shani's mum was devastated.

Shani refused to talk about it at first, but eventually explained that she was missing her dad and felt scared all the time. Her dad worked overseas for months at a time. Shani explained that she worried every night an intruder would come for her, her mum and her sister and that their dad wouldn't be home to protect them.

She explained that she tried to talk to her sister about how she felt more than once, but was always told she was being ridiculous.

Shani's mum took her to the GP and she was referred to a psychologist. Over time Shani revealed she felt angry with her sister and that the drawings helped her 'get her feelings out'.

Anxious behaviour isn't always problematic, though it can be disruptive. In a classroom setting, an anxious child might frequently seek their teacher's approval, or ask unnecessary questions to make sure they're doing everything right. They might struggle to concentrate and get out of their seat when they're meant to be working or they might chat to other kids who are then interrupted in their own work.

When anxiety is understood by parents and teachers, it's much easier to put the pieces of the puzzle together and get a clear picture of what's happening, and what to do about it.

For anxious kids of school age, communication between home and school helps them to bridge the divide between managing their anxiety in the comfort of home and in the less familiar, more unpredictable setting of a classroom.

## Teach anxious kids about their brain

When anxious kids understand what's happening in their brain it helps them to:

- understand what's at the heart of their anxiety
- recognise their symptoms
- make sense of how they think, feel and act when they're anxious
- think about their anxiety as a 'false alarm'
- know why they practise their management strategies
- have compassion for themselves when they're struggling
- feel empowered to move their anxiety to the background
- flourish.

## Explaining anxiety to kids

Kids and teens need to know what's going on in their brain when they're feeling anxious. It takes the mystery out of anxiety. Kids who understand anxiety learn to view it as a somewhat predictable process that serves the purpose of protecting them from danger.

Find a quiet time when they're relaxed, content and in the best frame of mind to take on new information. Encourage your child to approach the conversation with curiosity. If your anxious child is in primary school you could create a flow chart or poster together using colourful textas. This will serve as a colourful reminder of how amazing their brain is at keeping them safe and how it works hard sometimes to protect them from imagined danger. Older kids respond well to a conversation during which you make a few sketches and connections between the key points you're sharing with them. Some older kids will love creating a poster too.

Here's a script you can use with primary school-aged kids.

'So you know how you've been . . . having a lot of worries lately OR
getting overwhelmed quickly OR
feeling angry about issues that
    normally wouldn't bother you OR
feeling jumpy all the time OR
struggling to sit still and concentrate
    in class OR
not wanting to go to school OR
feeling too scared to go upstairs in
    the dark OR
feeling way too nervous to sleep
    over at a friend's house OR

_____

_____

_____

Well, lots of other kids feel exactly the same and there's a name for it; it's called anxiety.

There's an amazing part of your brain called the amygdala and its job is to keep you safe if there's a danger. It protects you by powering up your body so you can fight or run away really fast.

Sometimes your amygdala works a bit too hard to protect you even though you don't need it to. Your body gets all powered up for no reason and it can make you feel funny in the tummy like you do sometimes and/or:

teary

angry

worried

jumpy

sick

dizzy

like something's wrong

wanting to stay close to home

not wanting to be away from me for
    too long

_____

_____

It's not much fun when that happens, is it?

You know what, though? The best part of this is that you have an amazing brain that is always looking out for you. When it's being a bit over-protective, you can show your amygdala you're safe by breathing slowly and deeply. Focusing on what's happening now and learning new thinking skills will help too.'

You can add, 'The more you practise when you're feeling okay, the easier it will be to show your amygdala you're okay when it's being over-protective. I'd love to practise with you too; we can do it together.'

A great resource to help explain anxiety to younger kids, or anyone really, is a lovely illustrated book called *Hey Warrior* by Karen Young.

Here's a script you could use for older primary and secondary school kids:

'So you know how you keep getting an upset tummy and not wanting to go to school OR _____?
There's a really good explanation for why this keeps happening.

There's a part of your brain called the amygdala and its job is to protect you from danger. For some kids who have what's called anxiety, their amygdala senses danger even when they're safe. It's like when our smoke detector goes off when I burn the toast. It's a big reaction for a small problem. Sometimes the amygdala alarm goes off for no reason at all.

Lots of people have anxiety. It's really common. There'll be kids in your class who have anxiety too.

When your amygdala senses danger it switches on what's called the fight-or-flight response. That's your brain's way of powering you up to fight or flee the danger. Trouble is, when the body gets powered up and there's nothing to fight or escape from, it leaves your body feeling pretty awful.

When your brain goes into fight-or-flight mode, you're wanting to flee. In the case of school OR _____, you want to avoid it altogether.

OR When your brain goes into fight-or-flight mode you want to stand up to the 'danger'. When you're asked by your teacher to answer a question in class OR _____, your brain is gearing you up to protect you, which is why you start to feel angry.

Some of the changes that happen to power you up make your heart beat faster and you breathe more quickly so there's more oxygen going to your muscles. Some of the blood in your digestive system gets moved to your arms and legs so you can fight with more strength and run with more speed. That's why sometimes you feel like you're going to be sick. It can also make you feel dizzy and hot OR _____.

Anxiety makes it harder to concentrate and think clearly. No wonder you've been struggling a bit with school.

What's great is that you can show your amygdala you're safe. Breathing, mindfulness and using new thinking skills will help you to manage anxiety when it shows up.

We can make a plan so you can practise these skills. I'll support you every step of the way.'

## Other ideas to integrate into your explanation

Outside the heat of an anxious moment, let your child know that worry is the body's alarm system causing false alarms. Explain that this especially happens when a situation is new or unfamiliar. You could use the analogy of your child looking at situations through worry or anxiety glasses, finding all the possibilities that could go wrong; all the 'what ifs?'

It's also helpful to describe how when they're reading a scary story or watching a scary movie, they can feel scared even though they're not in danger. Help them make the link between those experiences and their experience of anxiety.

4

# Recognising anxiety in a child

Can you remember what it was like the first time you were faced with a spotty rash all over your new baby, or when you noticed lumps on the back of their neck or were managing their first fever? It's normal for us as parents to feel unsure and stressed, even anxious, when handling these situations for the first time. When it comes to parenting, there are so many firsts! There are firsts that make us feel excited and joyful, like smiles, gorgeous giggles and the much anticipated first words. Then there are the firsts that have us calling our wise friends for parenting advice, scheduling appointments at the GP or even consulting Dr Google (we advise against this, though – it's a strategy that frequently creates more anxiety than it relieves).

Over time, we become familiar and comfortable recognising a post-viral rash, or swollen lymph nodes due to a virus, and monitoring and managing a fever with less stress. We've 'been there, done that' and that experience enables us to recognise a familiar pattern or change, and act accordingly.

Unlike some of the physical ailments children experience, anxiety doesn't always conform to a particular pattern of signs and symptoms. It's different for different kids, and shows up in the social, emotional and academic aspects of their lives in a range of ways.

This makes anxiety tricky to recognise, unless you have experienced anxiety yourself. Anxious parents can usually identify signs of anxiety in their own children that might ordinarily be overlooked, for a while at least. Signs and symptoms of childhood anxiety can be similar to those experienced by adults.

In this chapter we're going to show you how to determine if your child's anxiety is a normal reaction to life events, and to recognise the signs and symptoms of different types of anxiety. We'll also explain when normal anxiety might be tipping over into becoming an anxiety disorder. Early recognition means early diagnosis and early intervention, helping to improve the quality of life for you, your child and your family. Take a few lovely deep breaths. Here we go.

## You're perfectly placed

Anxiety frequently goes undetected and, understandably, remains untreated, often for years. Half of anxious adults experienced symptoms as teenagers, so if you experienced anxiety when younger, you are well placed as a parent to recognise symptoms of it. Having done so, a visit to your GP will enable you to explore the nature of the symptoms together and plan your next move.

One large study of over 10 000 adolescents identified six years as the median age for the onset of anxiety symptoms.[1] This research revealed that despite the understanding that the first onset of anxiety and other mental disorders occurs in childhood or adolescence, it's common for treatment to occur years later.[2]

Take a moment to acknowledge the positive impact you will have on the trajectory of your child's mental health and wellbeing simply by reading and applying what you learn in this book. Your learning will help you to recognise the telltale signs of an anxiety disorder, if indeed there is one to identify, and take any necessary steps. Meeting with a professional doesn't mean there's a disorder that requires treatment. If there is, your child is ahead of the curve in terms of getting the help and support they need. Rest assured, if there is, you will adjust, and help is available for you too.

## The anxiety–calmness continuum

Anxiety exists on a continuum ranging from high calmness through to low calmness, mild anxiety through to high anxiety. This is different to the traditional view where anxiety is 'present' or 'absent'.[3] Noticing if your child is moving away from a more calm and relaxed persona to feeling more stressed, along with any accompanying behavioural change, is your cue to 'watch and wait' over time to see if these changes in fact point to anxiety.

Similarly, helping your child move in the direction of calmness helps buffer against stress.

## Behavioural clues

Young children often can't explain how they're thinking and feeling. Though kids get better at articulating how they're feeling as they get older, signs are often found in their actions. Sometimes behavioural clues are early signs of anxiety. At other times they become noticeable long after anxiety has become a concern.

Anxiety shows itself in different ways, which makes your role important. Most parents have an uncanny way of detecting even the most subtle changes in their child's mood, behaviour, voice, mannerisms, eating, attention and interactions. Trust yourself. You can also glean information from asking certain questions.

Child-anxiety expert associate professor Lynn Miller from Canada's University of British Columbia has developed a handy two-question test that parents can use to screen their kids for future anxiety disorders. Answers to the questions were found to be effective in identifying anxiety disorders in children 85 per cent of the time. The questions are:

1. Is your child more shy or anxious than other children their age?
2. Is your child more worried than other children their age?

Answering yes and yes to these questions doesn't mean your child has an anxiety disorder, but rather points to an increased possibility of one developing over time. This knowledge enables parents to bolster their child's resilience, thinking skills and self-regulation skills early.

## When is anxiety considered normal?

Anxiety is a normal reaction in stressful situations. At times, it can even be expected. Even when normal, anxiety can be distressing for a child and their parents. It's easy for a parent to worry that anxiety and distress are signs of bigger challenges to come. Fear not, this is the protective brain at work and eventually, as the threat passes, so too will the anxiety and the accompanying distress.

There are many circumstances that can evoke anxiety in kids, including:

- stressful events
- life changes
- transitions
- difficult experiences
- new or unfamiliar situations.[4]

There are also a range of developmental fears and anxieties that most children experience for a period of time. You may have seen some of these anxieties, such as separation anxiety or a fear of the dark.

Below is a guide to developmentally normal anxiety and fears in children and teenagers:

| Age | | Developmental fear and anxiety |
| --- | --- | --- |
| Early infancy | Within first weeks | Fear of losing physical contact with caregivers |
| | 0–6 months | Stimuli that stand out from the norm e.g. loud noise, sudden movement |
| Late infancy | 6–8 months | Shyness |
| | | Fear of strangers |
| Toddlerhood | 12–18 months | Separation anxiety |
| | 0–2 years | Loud noises, abrupt movement, thunderstorms, vacuum cleaners, popping balloons, people in costume (like Santa!) |
| | 2–3 years | Fear of thunder and lightning, fire, water, darkness, nightmares |
| | 3–4 years | The unfamiliar, scary noises, ghosts and goblins, monsters under the bed, burglars, fear of the dark, being alone in bed at night, strange noises, shadows on the wall in their bedroom |
| Early childhood | 4–6 years | Fear of death or dead people |
| | 5–6 years | Being separated from a parent, ghosts and monsters, the dark, being alone, getting lost, nightmares, thunder and lightning |
| Primary school age | 5–7 years | Fear of specific objects (animals, monsters, ghosts) |
| | | Fear of germs or getting a serious illness |
| | | Fear of natural disasters, fear of traumatic events e.g. getting burned, being hit by a car |
| | | School anxiety, performance anxiety |

*continues*

| Age | | Developmental fear and anxiety |
| --- | --- | --- |
| | 7–11 years | Being at home alone, something happening to their pets or people they love, being rejected or judged badly by their peers |
| Adolescence | 12–18 years | Rejection by peers |
| | | What their peers think of them |
| | | Someone they love getting sick or dying, how they're doing at school, what's going to happen after finishing high school, world events, intruders, natural disasters, fear of missing out[5] |

## When does normal anxiety become a disorder?

Anxiety that impairs the function and happiness of one child may in fact be quite well tolerated by another. Children who experience anxiety can also be happy much of the time.

A disorder is considered present when anxiety starts to interfere with a child's day-to-day functioning and quality of life. Watch for anxiety becoming debilitating or distressing and whether it becomes more severe, frequent and persistent over time.[6]

## When should I be worried?

Beyond Blue recommends erring on the side of caution, suggesting the more times you answer yes to any of the questions below, the more you need to consider talking over your observations with your child as well as with your GP.

• Have you noticed a change in behaviour?
• Is this change across multiple settings (home, school, work)?
• Is this behaviour occurring frequently?
• Has this been going on for more than two weeks?
• Is this change impacting on the young person's day-to-day life (for example, schoolwork or relationships)?[7]

## Signs and symptoms of anxiety

Many symptoms indicate anxiety; however, having those symptoms doesn't mean a child has an anxiety disorder.

Below we've included a list of signs and symptoms of anxiety disorders to look out for. Pay attention to how often your child is experiencing any signs of anxiety, the severity of their symptoms and over what period of time you've noticed these changes.

If you're concerned, make an appointment to ask the question of your health professional. Providing you can speak openly and honestly, you can choose to go to an initial appointment with or without your child. We recommend that you keep notes over time to track your child's signs and symptoms so that when you're with your health professional, you can accurately relay what's been happening. It's natural to feel worried and upset asking questions of your health professional about your child's mental health. Having a record of what's been going on helps you to paint a clear picture for a more accurate assessment of your child.

Signs and symptoms of anxiety are grouped according to their impact on children's emotions and physiology, behaviour and thinking.

## Emotionally and physically

It's common for anxiety symptoms to be physical given the changes that happen in the body when the fight-or-flight response is triggered. These can be worrying for kids. Many anxious kids worry that there's something physically 'wrong' with them that hasn't been identified. Teaching anxious kids what's happening in their brains and their bodies helps them to make sense of their symptoms and feelings.

Emotional and physical signs and symptoms of anxiety include:

- chest pain or discomfort
- discomfort or pain in the stomach; nausea

73

- dizziness, light-headedness, or unsteady feelings
- feeling foggy or detached from yourself
- feeling hot or cold
- feeling a lump in the throat or choking
- sleeplessness
- seeing spots
- headaches
- numbness or tingling
- diarrhoea
- tiredness
- rapid heart rate
- rapid breathing (hyperventilating), feelings of shortness of breath, or breath holding
- sweating
- trembling or shaking
- regularly crying over small problems
- angry outbursts
- often appearing nervous.

## Behaviour

It's hard for anxious kids to concentrate when they're feeling worried. It's equally challenging to concentrate when their body feels revved up like a race car that is stuck in the pits. It's no wonder anxiety shows in behaviours such as those listed below. Be mindful that some anxious kids can also be quiet and shy, while others may try to never put a foot out of line. It's easy to overlook anxiety in these kids. Behaviours indicating anxiety include:

- not participating in class, or being afraid to speak up or raise a hand
- excessive fear of making mistakes
- wanting to be 'perfect' in appearance and schoolwork
- refusing routine injections or visits to the dentist

- refusing to hang out with other kids or having few friends because of social fears
- not sleeping in their own bedroom or refusing to attend sleepovers
- refusing to go to school for any number of reasons (for example, an exam, performances, bullying, social situations)
- refusing to participate in sports, dance or other performance-related activities
- disliking taking risks or trying anything new
- avoiding situations they feel worried or scared about.

## Thinking

As the minds of anxious children are often on the lookout for threats and danger, they're thinking all the time: reflecting on events of the past, analysing situations and reactions from every angle, wondering what's going to happen next and worrying. If there was a 'Worrying Olympics', anxious kids would be gold medallists. Worrying and overthinking is a sign of anxiety.

While it's normal for all kids to worry, the minds of anxious kids generate worries that can overtake their thinking. Most of their worries seem irrational and inconsequential to the people who love and care for them, but in their minds the threats feel real.

Examples of worries experienced by anxious children include:

- I'm going to fail the test
- I might get it wrong
- Mum might forget to pick me up after school
- My teacher will yell at me and the kids will laugh
- That dog might bite me
- I could fall off my bike and embarrass myself
- I'll embarrass myself in front of my friends
- I'll get into trouble
- I could be sick at school
- Mum or Dad might die.

## Dependence

Anxious kids often seek reassurance. Their fight-or-flight response is triggered much of the time, causing them to feel threatened. Naturally, they want someone they trust to soothe them and reassure them they're okay. This dependence is part of the anxiety dance. If your child experiences anxiety, you may be familiar with some of these scenarios:

- asks for help with tasks they can do for themselves
- won't go to sleep without you or another trusted adult nearby
- asks, 'Will you do it for me?' or 'Will you tell them for me?'
- sees the dangerous or negative side of situations
- asks, 'Are you sure I won't get sick?'
- asks, 'Are you sure you'll be on time to pick me up?'
- asks parents to talk to teachers instead of doing so themselves
- doesn't want to be away from home for long or at all
- wants a parent to accompany them to parties and stay
- seeks ongoing reassurance about a worry (for example, that skin irritation is not cancer)
- frequently shares thoughts and worries
- shows dependent behaviour, including clinginess.

Under any of these anxious circumstances, deep, slow breathing will help your child to show their amygdala they're safe, eventually bringing their prefrontal cortex back online. In the meantime, avoid trying to use logic to persuade your child that their concerns are unfounded as this is unlikely to be helpful.

## Excess or extreme

As we mentioned earlier, anxious children can blow issues out of proportion, turning everyday occurrences into overwhelming problems. Do you recognise any of these scenarios?

- scared of the dark/dogs/being alone/tests
- expects the worst outcome
- has a knack for arriving at extreme conclusions from vague information
- has trouble falling asleep due to excessive worries about daily events, getting enough sleep, or staying asleep
- catastrophises a situation, imagining the worst-case scenario.

## Functioning

Children's anxiety can be a source of frustration for many parents. As we have discussed, when kids feel anxious they want to avoid the source of the anxiety. They can also feel anxious for one reason and then generally want to avoid anything that takes them out of their comfort zone. As we look at managing anxiety in coming chapters, we'll talk about helping anxious kids to be brave and take steps towards participating in activities, relationships and experiences that are important, including going to school and playing with their friends. Anxious kids don't have to wait until they feel perfectly calm to do what's important and function well. They can learn to turn down the volume on their anxiety and take it along for the ride.

Examples of how anxiety impacts children's functioning include:

- prefers to watch others rather than have a go
- doesn't want to get ready for school
- visits the school nurse often
- misses school
- finds it difficult or is unable to sit still for extended periods of time
- difficulty concentrating
- resists doing schoolwork
- is performing poorly at school

- experiences problems with friends and other peers
- is unable to do routine tasks without crying, tantrums or having continual reminders
- believes they can't cope or that it's safer to stay home
- doesn't get enough sleep or nutrition
- struggles academically
- withdraws socially
- struggles to balance reasonable demands such as homework or playing a sport.[8]

After reading the ways anxiety impacts on children, you may be considering the possibility that your child is indeed anxious. Alternatively, the examples might have confirmed what you already know: that your child is anxious. It's natural for either alternative to cause some parents stress.

It's hard as a parent to contemplate what a diagnosis of anxiety could mean for your child. Let us reassure you that if your child is diagnosed with an anxiety disorder, they're already on the pathway to the help and support they need to manage it. They're a step closer to understanding their thinking and how they feel, and the connection between the two and to living life in full colour.

You'll adjust to a new norm, and with health care professionals on your child's team you'll feel personally supported too. In addition to what you learn here, you'll further develop skills to assist your child to manage their anxiety in helpful, effective and sustainable ways.

You'll no longer be doing it alone or just with your partner; you'll be part of a team with your child's mental health at heart.

## Common types of anxiety

There are different anxiety disorders which have characteristic signs and symptoms. The most commonly diagnosed disorders in young people include generalised anxiety disorder, separation anxiety disorder, phobias, post-traumatic stress disorder (PTSD) and obsessive-compulsive disorder (OCD). Until the most recent publication of the *Diagnostic and Statistical Manual of Mental Disorders*, the *DSM–5*, OCD was included as an anxiety disorder but is now in a category of its own.

A discussion of PTSD is beyond the scope of this book, but let's take a look at the others now.

## Generalised anxiety disorder

The anxiety, constant worry and fears that a child with generalised anxiety disorder regularly feels can make it hard for them to meet the needs of their day. Avoidance is common to minimise feelings of anxiety that come with uncertainty or doing something new.

Generalised anxiety disorder makes it hard for children to see situations and events for what they are; their thoughts usually focus on negative possibilities and outcomes. They'll seek comfort in the reassurance from a parent or trusted adult that they're okay, that what they're worried about isn't cause for concern and that the catastrophes they predict won't happen.

## Separation anxiety disorder

Separation anxiety disorder is developmentally normal between a child's first birthday and around eighteen months to two years of age. Many children will experience difficulty separating from their parent (sometimes one parent more than the other) at the start of kinder or even at the beginning of primary school. Most of these difficulties resolve quickly, but separation anxiety can become an ongoing challenge for some families.

Some children fear that something awful will happen to them or someone they love, usually their parent, while they're separated. Younger children can struggle to understand why their parent (or other much loved adult) is leaving them at all and if they'll ever return. These fears underlie separation anxiety disorder.

Children experiencing anxiety of this type feel distressed at being separated and so it makes sense that they'll avoid it at all costs. Hence the tears, the pleading, the clinginess and the unwillingness to say farewell.

Separation anxiety disorder can be diagnosed when distress on separation does not naturally reduce after around two years of age and the intensity of the child's anxiety remains severe.[9]

The anxiety can extend to not wanting to go to school, complaining of tummy aches and sickness to avoid a separation, distress at staying overnight at a friend's house or worry about going on school camp. Children experiencing separation anxiety can also experience vomiting and diarrhoea.[10]

## Phobias

We've all experienced fear. It's natural to feel fear when our safety is threatened. Sometimes we deliberately put ourselves in a situation that makes us scared and anxious, like bungee jumping or skydiving. We can experience fear in these situations and yet make a conscious choice to go ahead and jump, knowing deep down that the chances of us getting seriously hurt are small and are outweighed by the thrill of the experience.

Kids do the same; they'll approach a skate bowl with more confidence than they should at times, they'll pick up insects adults might avoid, they'll jump off a cliff ledge into water or they'll attempt new tricks on the trampoline with confidence. They might experience fear under some of these circumstances but take the 'leap' anyway.

Phobias are different. When a kid has a phobia, their aversion to a particular type of activity, animal or situation is exaggerated and irrational. They hold a genuine belief that what they're scared of poses a genuine and serious threat to their safety. In anticipation of the specific object, animal or situation, kids with phobias experience extreme anxiety and will avoid exposure as if their life depended on it. This can cause panic attacks – a short-lived episode of intense anxiety – for some kids.

Common children's phobias include:

- animals such as dogs or birds
- insects or spiders
- the dark
- loud noises
- storms
- clowns, masks or unusual-looking people
- blood
- illness
- injections.

## Social anxiety disorder

Kids diagnosed with social anxiety disorder, sometimes called social phobia, struggle with social situations of any kind. Avoidance is central to the behaviour patterns in children with this diagnosis. When kids with social anxiety disorder are around other people, their thoughts turn to questions about how they're being seen or judged. They're afraid of embarrassing themselves, being rejected and/or being thought of as stupid, ugly or strange.

It's difficult for children with social anxiety disorder to see situations for what they are: a time to relax and enjoy themselves. They want to, but their anxiety makes hanging out with friends difficult, let alone meeting new people, being the centre of attention or performing in a public setting.

Kids with social anxiety disorder deal with their anxiety by staying in their comfort zone whenever possible. The signs and symptoms of this type of anxiety are related to avoiding other people and feeling distressed when they unavoidably find themselves in a social setting. Their distress at presenting in front of their class or meeting new people is out of proportion to what other children are typically experiencing under the same circumstances.

More girls than boys are diagnosed with social anxiety disorder. The median age of onset is 14.5 years.[11]

## Obsessive-compulsive disorder (OCD)

Have you ever double or triple checked you've turned off the iron, heater or stove? Perhaps you've rechecked the doors are locked before heading off to bed at night, knowing you've already locked everything up only minutes before? Maybe you've checked your bag for your boarding pass more than once on your way to your departure gate at the airport.

Many of us have done one or all of these at some time or another. We get a nagging feeling that makes us uncomfortable and an extra check is all we need to feel reassured everything is in order. Often the reason we recheck is because our mind was wandering when we flicked the switch on an appliance, locked the door or checked for our ticket the first time.

Compulsions including checking and rechecking, ordering items and handwashing are examples of symptoms of obsessive-compulsive disorder, or OCD.

OCD, as the name suggests, has symptoms falling into two categories: obsessions and compulsions. Obsessions are defined as recurrent and persistent thoughts, urges or impulses that are intrusive and unwanted, causing distress. Compulsions conform to rigid rules and include behaviours and mental acts such as repetitive handwashing, ordering, checking, counting, praying, repeating words silently or repeatedly telling a parent something. Compulsions are performed to counteract or neutralise the obsession, relieving the feelings of anxiety.[12]

Common obsessions in young people include:

- fear of germs
- violent thoughts, including thoughts about hurting themselves or someone they love
- imagining frightening or rude mental pictures

- fear of doing something wrong in the future
- fear of having already done something wrong
- self-doubt
- the need for items to be orderly, even or symmetrical.[13]

Common compulsions include:

- checking
- counting
- washing hands
- doing work all over again to ensure it's 'perfect'
- making steps, clicks of a light switch, turns of a handle or other actions 'even'
- asking questions for reassurance
- confessing thoughts
- collecting or hoarding items
- touching items in a particular sequence or a certain number of times
- keeping to a strict routine.

Hoarding is a common sign of OCD in children, more so for girls than boys. Children can also hear an inner voice ordering them to perform rituals and other compulsions. They can be indecisive, unusually slow in everyday activities and feel greatly relieved when a compulsion has been completed.[14]

OCD is diagnosed when obsessions and compulsions:

- cause unhappiness and distress
- get in the way of daily functioning and participation in normal activities
- take up a great deal of time
- interfere with normal everyday routines
- affect family relationships.

The average age of onset of OCD for young people is between 7.5 years and 12.5 years of age. Three boys experience OCD for every two girls, though for older adolescents, slightly more girls than boys are diagnosed.[15] Similar to other types of anxiety, OCD is treatable. Kids with OCD can learn to understand and manage their symptoms and live a rich and full life.

## What does anxiety look like at school?

Anxious kids frequently find school difficult. Symptoms can become more frequent and more distressing during the school term compared with how they appear during school holiday breaks. As the end of the holidays approaches, anxious kids often start to think about their imminent return to school and the familiar feeling of anxiety begins to build.

Here are some signs to look out for at school that could indicate a child is anxious:

- having difficulty concentrating
- making frequent visits to the school nurse
- often being distracted
- being a perfectionist
- making careless mistakes
- being impulsive
- being unable to sit still
- reducing their involvement in classroom activities
- having excess energy
- being fidgety
- loving details
- avoiding the spotlight
- freezing when called upon to answer a question.

School timetables and routines offer a degree of certainty for anxious kids but much about a school day is unpredictable. Within their classroom, an anxious child can be challenged by a variety of influences including the actions of their peers, impromptu questions from their teacher, the complexity of their work and/or their environment. Heavily decorated classrooms can affect attention and learning and increase anxiety for some children.

Outside of the classroom, uncertainty abounds. Anxious children can be affected by crowds of students, noise and the unpredictability of social interactions, to name a few variables. Schools with quiet places for children to enjoy respite are few and far between.

We know of one nurse new to a primary school who quickly discovered anxious children liked to visit the sick bay to escape the bustle of the schoolyard. She affectionately called them her 'frequent flyers' and always offered them a quiet place to rest. She understood that anxious children need a space at school where they feel relaxed enough for their nervous system to begin to calm down.

# Part 3

# Parenting anxious kids

If anxiety is to be managed and minimised in the long term, children and young people need the tools and skills to be able to manage their own states. This part will focus on the parenting style that's best suited to helping this process. It can't be stressed too much that parents are in the best possible position to assist their children to manage anxiousness. This means that parents should be cognisant of the physiology of anxiety so that they can pass on key understandings to their children. Such knowledge will also help parents feel more comfortable and confident dealing with feelings of anxiousness and worry. Parents also need to be aware of the behaviours that they project both when they are stressed and also when their children become anxious. This type of self-awareness is a precursor to parents modelling effective ways of responding and managing stress for their children.

It's our firm belief that children and teenagers shouldn't be sheltered from the challenges and expectations of everyday life. Their anxiety needs to be factored in, but should not excuse kids from participating in normal daily events. The promotion of real independence and resilience needs to be at the heart of parenting anxious kids. Both are traits that will help kids to function effectively, and eventually feel less anxious over time. This section of the book will show you how to develop independence and resilience in your kids.

# 5

# Modelling

So you have an anxious child. How you respond to their anxiousness will go a long way to either assisting or hindering their self-management. The key to working with children is not to endeavour to cure them of anxiety, but to assist them to recognise it, to understand its causes and then to manage it (put it into the background) while they get on with their lives. So how do you respond to their anxiousness? Do you respond calmly and methodically, or does their anxiety agitate you and make you tense? In this chapter we will show you how to respond appropriately when kids are anxious, and discuss the impact of modelling on children.

## The impact of modelling

Children are primed to copy. They copy our words, our actions, even our attitudes. If that sounds a little freaky, spend some time around a two-year-old and you'll be reminded that mimicry is their primary learning mode.

It's not just two-year-olds who copy. Kids of all ages are close observers of the behaviours of their parents and other people they spend time with. Children and teenagers see their parents at very close quarters. They witness many of our happiest moments and so see us at our best. They also see us under stress when life doesn't go well and, importantly, see how we handle it – how we react to our loved ones and how we approach challenging situations. They see if we avoid them or if we take a big breath and tackle challenges full on. These are tremendously important lessons that kids learn. It's the behaviours they witness when we're under stress that usually have the greatest impact on children. Adult behaviours when accompanied by high emotion are generally most memorable for children. If we catastrophise and blow issues out of all proportion, there is every likelihood that children will see catastrophising as a normal response mechanism. When we respond thoughtfully and calmly to a difficult situation, we show our kids how to respond in similar ways.

## Michael's story

After a day spent with my friend's family we were getting ready for a group photo, but Mr Thirteen suddenly became reluctant. I playfully placed him in a headlock and good-naturedly pulled him in for the shot. The photo was taken and we all had a laugh about it. I quietly congratulated myself for winning the young boy over. Two minutes later all hell broke loose. The thirteen-year-old had grabbed his younger brother in a headlock and dragged him to the ground. And he didn't let go. His father yelled at him to stop, but Mr Thirteen wasn't listening. It took some very physical intervention from his dad to bring the wrestling to a halt. The previously harmonious scene was gone, replaced by angst and anger from parents and kids. I'd done the wrong thing when I grabbed Mr Thirteen in a playful headlock. Even though it was meant in jest, it gave

Mr Thirteen permission to do the same to his younger brother.

His action wasn't in the spirit of playfulness as mine had been. It was malicious, but that didn't alter the fact that I gave him permission to place his brother in a headlock by doing the same to him.

Parents not only teach kids how to behave through our modelling, our own actions give kids permission to behave in those same ways. In fact, we give our kids permission all the time through our behaviour. When we overreact, catastrophise or make excuses we give our kids permission to do the same. The permission is implicit rather than explicit. We don't actually say to our kids, 'It's okay to jump to conclusions and think that the world is falling apart. Go on, stress yourself out with your ramblings!' But our behaviour speaks louder than our words.

## Using the psychology of permission positively

Conversely, we give kids permission to be calm, rational and thoughtful when we behave in those ways. Our behaviour under stress shows them how to regulate their emotions and actions. That's why modelling is such a powerful shaper of children's behaviour.

And it's even more impactful when a child holds their parent in high regard. That makes the early and middle years of childhood, when parents most influence their kids' lives, the ages when modelling is of paramount importance.

## What permission means as a parent

It could be argued that parenthood is the great maturing agent of our time. In an era when young people seem stuck in a long, drawn-out adolescence, the birth of their first child is an introduction to selflessness and responsibility. Apart from the fact that new parents become instantly responsible for the upbringing of someone apart from themselves, the fact that the minutiae of their behaviour is being watched and copied by another is a game changer.

The realisation that their behaviour provides their children with permission to act in similar ways is the scariest thing. Quite simply, parents, in particular, and adults, in general, need to be mindful about how we behave when kids are around. We don't want to put a dampener on a person's playfulness, spontaneity and sense of individuality, but when kids are around, you have to think and be smart about how you behave.

## Displaying positive behaviours

There are three main behaviours that parents can use to assist their children to better manage their anxiety: responding empathetically rather than reacting emotionally to stressful situations; using healthy coping mechanisms when life becomes difficult; and developing a healthy lifestyle to minimise anxiety and its impact.

## 1. Responding empathetically

Think of a time when your child came to you very upset about something done to them. Perhaps they'd been unfairly treated by a teacher, or they'd been told off by a coach in front of the team, or they had been ostracised by an insensitive peer group. Regardless, you may have felt angry at what your child experienced, and perhaps even felt the need for retaliation. Think what you did next. Did you react angrily? Did you take charge and look to rescue your child from this difficult situation? Did you relinquish all emotion and ignore your child's emotional needs? Alternatively, did you manage to take a breath, stay calm and give yourself a chance to think things through? Let's look a little further at each and work out which of the four approaches are most appropriate if we want to help kids better manage their anxieties and worries.

### React

It's the most natural thing in the world to react emotionally when our kids are in trouble. It's akin to the fight-or-flight response, in which our default is to act quickly when trouble is looming. We don't think straight when we react emotionally. We tend to overreact, exaggerate a situation or imagine the worst possible scenario. Often people make decisions they later regret when they react emotionally to an event, which is a sure sign that although their reaction may have made them feel better at the time, it didn't achieve great results.

### Rescue

Imagine your child is extremely stressed by the prospect of going to school the next day as they know they are going to sit a test they are not prepared for. They work themselves into a lather, and then begin blaming the teacher for not giving them enough time to prepare. 'It's totally not fair. It's just a waste of time even going to school because I'm going to fail. Then my teacher will hate me even more.' They start to push the 'not fair' and 'teacher hates me' buttons, which make you feel guilty. Despite knowing deep down that your child should go to school, you start to doubt your tough stance, so you let them take the day off . . . 'Just this once.' You've rescued your child from facing the music, and by the looks of things they feel better already because they've suddenly calmed down. Yes, it's easy to rescue children from situations that cause them real or feigned anxiety, but in the long run all a child learns is that if a situation upsets them, it's better to avoid it than put up with the discomfort of having a go, and possibly surprising themselves that the test – or whatever it is they are not looking forward to – isn't so bad after all.

### Relinquish

'Dad, the coach won't play me in the centre. He keeps putting me in the backline and I'm crap playing there.'

'Son, you've got to play where the coach puts you. He's got his reasons for playing you in the backline.'

'Thanks for nothing, Dad!' The boy storms off to his bedroom, slamming the door behind him.

This dad focused on his son's behaviours and forgot to focus on his emotions. In effect, he relinquished his attention to his son's immediate emotional needs and focused instead on a different picture, which was fitting in with the team. When kids are upset, stressed or anxious they invariably narrow their vision to themselves, and have difficulty seeing past their own navel.

### Respond

Let's play the above scenario out again but let's see what happens if the father focuses on his son's emotional needs first.

'Dad, the coach won't play me in the centre. He keeps putting me in the backline and I'm crap playing there.'

'Son, it sounds like you're pretty annoyed by the whole thing.'

'Yep, I hate footy at the moment. I just can't get a kick.'

'Is it the position you're playing or that you're just having a bad trot?'

'I dunno. None of the other kids kick it to me . . .'

The conversation headed down a completely different path when this father took an empathetic approach and focused on his son's emotions. He responded in a way that met his son's needs – that is, feeling understood. He was then able to steer the conversation down a path where his son began to open up and talk about what was really bothering him.

The above examples focus on the approaches parents use to address children's stresses and worries. But we also need to be mindful of how we respond to our own stresses and anxieties when kids are around. If we react emotionally, if we avoid difficult situations or ignore how we feel and go on with life regardless, we are teaching our kids to do the same. We want kids to respond rationally and thoughtfully when they feel anxious or stressed. We want them to be able to step back a little, take a breath and calm their amygdala before they respond.

## 2. Coping out loud

The good, the bad and the ugly are all on display when we're parents. You can't hide it from kids. If you're a pessimist, it will show through in the way you approach difficult situations. If you're the sort of person who leaps before they look, the kids will see that too. If you're a panic merchant who turns molehills into mountains, then kids can't help but notice that. Conversely, kids can see us manage potentially anxious moments with calm and aplomb, if this is the approach we choose to take. Given this, it makes sense to amplify the healthy ways of managing difficulties so that children and teenagers can see how healthy adults cope with their worries and difficulties.

Here are some healthy ways to manage your stresses that you can model for your kids to see.

### Catch yourself ruminating

Perversely, even though we know that worry is not good for us, when faced with a difficult situation we worry about it continually because we think it will help by maintaining feelings of control. When you catch yourself ruminating about future events, ask, 'Is overthinking it going to help me solve this problem?' If not, change your thinking to something more useful, such as mentally rehearsing a successful approach to the situation.

### Challenge your thinking (about your worries)

Most people who experience generalised anxiety will either overestimate the likelihood of something bad happening or underestimate their ability to cope. An event will be 'an absolute disaster' or they will 'have a nervous breakdown' if they have to attend. Challenge these worrying thoughts by questioning their validity. 'How likely is it that this will occur?' Recall past experiences that provide evidence you will be able to cope.

### Exercise

Exercise is a healthy way of coping with feelings of anxiety. When you feel overwhelmed by anxiety do something physical such as going for a brisk walk, playing with the kids or going to the gym. Discuss with your kids why you are exercising and let them know the positive impact it has on you.

### Distract yourself

Rather than brood about your worries, which seems only to make them bigger, do something to take your mind off them for a time. Play a game, watch some TV, play a video game or go out – do something to distract yourself. Show your kids that self-distraction is healthy and usually provides a sense of perspective. It also prevents you from amplifying possible future experiences and blowing them out of all proportion.

### Relax

When you're anxious you generally have high levels of arousal, which means that it can be hard to relax and calm down. You may notice that you can't sit still, that you keep tapping your leg or constantly fidget. This makes relaxation difficult, even though it is perhaps the most helpful thing you can do. If this is the case, try techniques such as progressive muscle relaxation or mindfulness (see Chapter 11) to help turn the mental chatter down and maintain feelings of calm.

Here are some coping scripts for you to use in front of your kids:

'I'm feeling anxious right now; I'm not sure why but it doesn't matter. I'm going to stop for five belly breaths, which I know always helps.'

'I can't give you my full attention at the moment because I'm trying to complete this online form and I'm so frustrated by it. I'm going to go outside for five minutes of walking and fresh air before I try again. I'll come and find you when I've finished. Okay?'

'My mind keeps fast-forwarding to the presentation I have to give tomorrow at work. I'm feeling nervous. I'm going to sit in the lounge room and do a mindfulness exercise to bring my thinking back to the present.'

'There's so much to do to pack for our holiday. I'm taking a few minutes to notice everything I can hear so I can be more mindful and focus on what I need to do. Then I'm going to make a list and do one thing at a time to make sure we have everything we need.'

## 3. Healthy lifestyle

Psychologist and speaker Andrew Fuller is fond of telling audiences that the job of parents is to teach their kids to live life well. This is a lovely turn of phrase which helps us focus on the important parts of parenting. It's a reminder that not only our language and attitudes are on show for kids to copy, but our lifestyle too. A healthy lifestyle is one that includes good mental and physical health habits. Sleep, exercise, use of alcohol and how we relate to each other all impact on mental health and anxiety. Other parts of this book will explore healthy lifestyle factors that help minimise anxiety and maximise children's abilities to lead happy lives even when anxiety looms. For now, it's worth remembering that children and young people will generally take the lead of their parents, so consider the type of lifestyle that you have on show for your children to mimic.

# 6

# Responding to a child's anxious moment

In the previous chapter we discussed the impact of modelling on the approach kids take to managing their own anxiety. We covered four common responses that parents can have – react, rescue, relinquish or respond. In this chapter we'd like to further explore how you can respond effectively to a child when they are experiencing a significant anxiety moment, so that they feel they are being heard and understood, and, significantly, so you can help them stay calm rather than be overwhelmed or panicked by their thoughts and feelings.

We will introduce you to two frameworks that can work simultaneously. First, the SOBER framework focuses on you as a parent so you can respond effectively. The second framework – the Anxiety Response Plan – shows you how to respond to an anxious child.

Stay SOBER – well, of course, right?

Anxiety is contagious, so it's easy for your own stress and worry to get in the way when responding to your anxious child. Remembering what's important in the moment is so much harder when your own anxiety shows up because it interferes with decision-making. That's why we're so fond of the easy-to-remember acronym SOBER.[1]

**S**  Stop

**O**  Observe

**B**  Breathe

**E**  Expand

**R**  Respond

## Stop

Multi-tasking can play a big part in parenting. Of an evening in a typical home there's dinner to prepare and cook, maybe readers to listen to or homework to help with. There might be washing to hang out, bills to pay, emails to reply to and stories from the day to share. Many of these tasks are done at the same time. All families fall into these patterns at one time or another. It can so often feel like there just aren't enough hours in the day to get everything done.

We get it, and we've been there too. But what we can tell you is that multi-tasking is a misnomer. It's not actually possible to do any two high-level thinking tasks at once. It feels like multi-tasking but it's actually task switching. It happens so fast it feels like two things are happening at once. It's like toggling quickly between two tabs open on your computer screen.

When it comes to parenting an anxious child, they need your full attention during anxious times. By providing them with your undivided attention, you're in a much better position to respond in the helpful new ways you're learning here. You don't necessarily need to drop everything the instant your child needs you; it's okay to say that you're in the middle of doing something but that you'll be with them in a moment. That way, when you are with them, it's easier to be present and really listen. Multi-tasking also increases stress, and you probably already have enough of that too.

## Observe

This is your opportunity to take in what's actually happening. To be the observer. Observing the situation for what it is. It's a simple idea, but not always easy. What's your child doing at the moment? What is their behaviour telling you? What are you thinking about as this scene unfolds before you? Are you annoyed that this is happening again? Are you feeling impatient, wanting to step in and fix it so that it's over with? Or are you feeling a sense of sadness that your child is suffering in this moment? Being able to take a mental step back and observe what's going on under these circumstances is something that will take time. Please be compassionate and patient with yourself.

## Breathe

Breathing deeply and slowly is the one way the relaxation response can be initiated and the fight-or-flight response can be dialled down. Taking a moment for a few breaths here is your way to settle any of your own stress and anxiety so that you're in a good frame of mind to thoughtfully respond to what's happening.

## Expand

This next part of the SOBER approach refers to expanding your awareness to the possibilities in the moment. Where are you? What's happening next? Are you in the best position to respond in the way you would like? If you're already running late for an appointment and anxiety shows up, how can you respond in a way that keeps everyone moving forward without revisiting past habits of avoidance and reassurance? What are your options?

## Respond

The very first sentence to pass your lips as a parent responding to an anxious child needs to be one of validation. This is your chance to say, 'I get it.'

Babies cry to let their parents know they need something. The needs of some babies become quite predictable, and so are easier to recognise and meet, as they follow the feed, play, sleep cycle, with nappy changes thrown into the mix. Their behaviour, in the form of crying, is a message expressing, among other things, 'I'm hungry', 'I'm tired', 'I'm uncomfortable' or 'I need hugs'. The same holds true for anxious children. Their actions are a message to you as the parent.

They could be frustrated, angry, teary, keen to share their worries or wanting to avoid an anxiety-provoking situation. All of these are signs that they're anxious, and what they need first and foremost is for you to recognise they're in need and then communicate to them that their message is received. Here are some things you could say:

'I can see you're feeling worried about going to the party.'

'Thanks for telling me you're feeling so nervous about the test. I get it.'

'Oh I get it, you're having the thought that no reply to your text means you must have done something wrong.'

'I hear you.'

'I know what that feels like.'

All of these responses are examples of responding with empathy.

Dr Brené Brown explains how empathy is feeling *with* people. It's about tapping into the same feeling within yourself and letting the other person know you understand because you've been there too (without turning the conversation onto yourself).

This is what anxious kids need from their parents. And if you're not sure what to say in the moment, you can simply start by saying, 'I'm so glad you told me.'

It may take you a little practice to remember to put these thinking skills into play when you're responding to your child's anxiety. That's perfectly fine. You're human, and these situations can be upsetting and stressful. Eventually, though, it will become more automatic. Each time you practise using SOBER, you're retraining your brain to respond in this helpful way.

## The big picture

*'The most important thing is remembering the most important thing.'*

— Suzuki Roshi

Anxiety is unpredictable, and can show up at the most inconvenient times. When children are anxious and not wanting to go to school, to a party, to visit a friend, to the shopping centre or even to training for their favourite sport, it can bring about extreme frustration for parents. Remember to be kind and compassionate to yourself if you've had some unhelpful thoughts of your own.

For anxious kids, the flight part of their fight-or-flight response is at play here. Leaving the house to go to certain places, or sometimes just to go anywhere, can set off their internal alarm, and avoidance – taking flight – feels like the safest option.

Because their brains are working so hard to keep them out of danger, they can struggle to see the woods for the trees. Their vision becomes narrowly focused and they can lose sight of what really matters to them.

## Sarah's story

Sarah found a part-time job at the local bakery as soon as she was fifteen. She was highly motivated by her dream of travelling around Europe with her bestie after they finished Year Twelve, and so she saved half of everything she earned.

Sarah's anxiety had been diagnosed by the family GP when she was twelve. A proactive young person, Sarah managed her anxiety well through daily meditation and regular exercise, but as birthdays came and went, with increasing school and social pressures, she began to find it harder to get going in the mornings. She started talking about resigning from her job.

Sarah's parents didn't know at the time how powerful their response was to Sarah's musings about quitting. By reminding her why she found the job in the first place, and how amazing her overseas adventures would be, they were able to spark in Sarah the willingness to keep her job with the constant reminder that it was part of a bigger plan.

They took Sarah to a travel agent to pick up some brochures so she could cover the walls of her bedroom with glossy pictures of the places she planned to visit. This way she would be constantly reminded to keep moving towards her goal, despite her anxiety.

## Plan your response

Knowing in advance how you'd like to respond to a child who is panicking or working themselves up emotionally to the point of hyperventilation can be extremely helpful. We have found the approach outlined in the table later in the chapter to be useful in calming kids down when they've become overwhelmed with worry.

## Recognition

Perhaps the hardest part of this process for parents is recognising that a child is anxious or panicking. It helps when you know the types of situations that are likely to trigger an anxiety attack. If tackling new subjects or topics at school have been the cause of anxiety in the past, then it will come as no surprise if your child is reluctant to go to school at the start of the year. It also helps to know how your child's anxiety typically presents – anger, tears, avoidance and going sullen or quiet are a few possible behaviours. You can become so busy at times that you miss the obvious signs. Alternatively, kids who experience anxiety might surprise you when a situation or event that hasn't caused worry in the past begins to cause anxiety for the first time. Recognition grows easier as you become more adept at tuning in to your child's wavelength.

## Validation

Above all else, kids want understanding when they are anxious. You don't have to fix their problem, but you do have to show that you understand they are anxious. 'Ahhhh' statements are a brilliant way to validate how your child is feeling. Repeating back what you're hearing shows you're listening and trying to understand. It's also a great way to help your child develop a more nuanced emotional vocabulary:

'Ahhhh, you're feeling anxious right now . . .'

'Ahhhh, you're having one of those "I might mess it up" ideas . . .'

'Ahhhh, you're feeling disappointed that it didn't work out for you . . .'

## Breathe

Just as it's important that you take some deep breaths when your child is anxious to prevent you feeling the same way, we highly recommend that you prompt your child to breathe. If they are familiar with deep-breathing techniques, then quietly remind them to take some big breaths. If deep breathing is new, or your child is struggling to calm down, then take some deep breaths together by suggesting, 'Come on, let's take three big breaths.'

## Attention

A child in the midst of a panic attack or who is overwhelmed by anxiousness invariably has their thoughts firmly planted in the future, worrying about an event or situation that hasn't happened yet. Bring their attention back to the present through their sense of touch, sight, hearing or feeling.

## Action

When a child or teen has calmed down, guide them towards the action that matters. If it's a test at school that's brought on an anxious moment, then help your child make plans to tackle the test as well as they can. Talk through how they can prepare. Remind them that they can only do their best, and that you would be happy with that. Do as much as you can to relieve the pressure and stress from the situation but don't allow avoidance to be an option.

| Anxiety Response Plan | |
|---|---|
| 1. Recognise your child's anxiety:<br>    • Know the triggers, e.g. an upcoming test, having to give a speech, meeting new friends<br>    • Know how it presents, e.g. anger, tears, avoidance. | Recognition |
| 2. Validate how they feel:<br>    • Use 'Ahhhh' statements<br>    • Match your response<br>    • Build their environment vocabulary. | Validation |

| | |
|---|---|
| 3. Prompt deep, slow breathing:<br>&bull; Remind them to breathe, e.g. 'Let's take three deep breaths together.' | Breathe |
| 4. Bring their attention back to the present:<br>&bull; Use senses to shift their attention e.g. 'What can you see, hear and touch?'<br>&bull; Get them moving, e.g. mindful walking. | Attention |
| 5. Guide them to take action towards what matters:<br>&bull; Remind them of what's important e.g. school success, playing with friends, enjoying sport<br>&bull; Recommit to successful action. | Action |

## A word about tolerating discomfort

Though not a distinct step in the Anxiety Response Plan, supporting your anxious child to tolerate their discomfort is an approach you can incorporate into your validation of their experience of anxiety in the moment.

Kids tolerate discomfort all the time. They just don't realise it. Tolerating discomfort is a skill. It's helpful to think of it as a 'muscle' that gets stronger with training. Each time they successfully tolerate discomfort, they're reinforcing their ability to do so and cementing the knowledge that they always come out the other side intact.

Naming a feeling and tolerating the discomfort of that feeling will help them move through it sooner than they would had they pushed it aside.

Tolerating discomfort is a willingness to sit with an uncomfortable or emotionally painful feeling. Opportunities for practice are plentiful and are found in situations like these when a child is:

- feeling hungry
- feeling thirsty
- wanting something they can't have
- having to end screen time

- contributing to household chores
- missing out on a job interview
- asking someone on a date
- excluded from a party.

Tolerating discomfort doesn't mean toughing it out. It's about teaching your anxious child to notice how they're feeling, how to name their emotions, and practise acceptance of how they feel in that moment. All with the knowledge that what they're experiencing is temporary and that they're lovingly supported by a warm and comforting parent. Couple tolerating discomfort with social rewards (such as words of praise or a shared fun activity) for coping behaviours and you're helping to strengthen effective coping skills.

## Reducing anxiety through social storytelling

Kids who are anxious by nature generally dislike change and feel uncomfortable when confronted with new events, new social situations and new groups of people. You may notice they become a little more agitated as they approach the start of the school year and realise that they'll have to adjust to a change of teacher, make new friends and possibly go to a different part of the school. Alternatively, you may notice a child making last-minute excuses about starting jazz ballet as initial excitement is replaced by nerves and tension as the date comes closer. Relatively mild agitation and uncertainty at the prospect of approaching new events or situations is generally greatly elevated when a child or teen is feeling particularly vulnerable, or has a lot going on in their lives.

The best way to avoid last-minute anxiety is to provide an anxious child with as much information as possible, helping them prepare for the event ahead. We recommend that you develop the habit of walking your child through new scenarios to help them feel comfortable and in control. Be as vivid as you possibly can, cuing them about how they may prepare themselves for new scenarios. Kate Johnson, founder of Spectrum Journeys, an organisation assisting parents of children with autism, calls this type of preparation 'social storytelling'. Johnson believes that for children on the autism spectrum to function effectively, parents and teachers must first help them manage their anxiety. Social storytelling is a powerful way of assisting children with autism to manage new situations and events. It's not just children on the spectrum who benefit. Anyone who experiences anxiety will benefit when a loving adult calmly walks them through a new situation or event. Here's an example:

'Alexander, when you go to Noah's party you know there'll be children there who you don't know. You need to be prepared for that. Maybe you can think about what to say when you meet some new friends. I'll take you there, but I'll only stay for a few minutes till you settle in. Then I'm going to leave because I haven't been invited. You need to be prepared for that. Okay? You know Noah's mum, so you can go to her if you feel like you want to take a break. There'll probably be some party games. You may not want to join in all of them but I think you should play at least one. Okay? You may want to think about the games you want to play before you go. Remember, your dad will pick you up. He'll meet you inside the house. Okay? If he's not there on time just wait because he may have been caught in traffic.'

## Be prepared to ease the load

Many kids who experience anxiety are also highly driven, achievement-oriented students. It's easy for a young person to fill their schedule with challenging learning tasks and activities so that they become overwhelmed. Year Twelve? Yes. Football? Yes. Part-time job? Of course. School play? Why not? Charity run? Definitely. When a highly motivated child or young person is stretched it often only takes one extra activity added to their schedule, an illness or a small downturn in their school marks for their anxiety to run amok. Suddenly everything makes them anxious. They stress about football; they fret about their marks; they regret taking that job; they have self-doubt about the school play; and they can't even contemplate participating in the charity run. It's not that any one activity alone causes stress, but the sheer volume of activities when combined can make it seem that everything is causing anxiety. At this point it's best for parents to look for ways to ease the load. Help them reconfigure their schedule, discussing the activities that they should abandon or put on hold. Consider giving them less independence and increasing the amount of help you provide with many of their everyday tasks. Also consider decreasing the jobs they do around the house in an effort to give them some time for relaxation and to prevent overload, which is frequently behind a great deal of anxiety.

## A final word

Anxious kids often need help to take a metaphorical step back and perceive the bigger picture. They need someone to assist them to see things as they are, rather than through the clouded lens of anxiety. The bigger picture is often very clear to you, as the parent of an anxious child; if it's not, take some time to talk to your child or teen about what's really important to them.

As you gain a clear picture of what's happening in the moment with your anxious child, part of your role will be to consider what's standing in the way of them moving forward, to help them lessen any load that may weigh them down and encourage them to take life one small step at a time.

# 7

# Parenting for resilience and independence

Resilience and independence are popular buzzwords at the moment. So prolific are these terms, in fact, that their meanings and significance seem to have been lost. These terms are not interchangeable but they are closely linked to each other; you can't have one without the other. A child can't be resilient if they are dependent on others. Similarly, a child needs to be resilient if they are to become independent. The path to gaining independence can be a rocky road to travel along, so resilience and independence go hand in hand.

Definitions of resilience abound. Psychologist and speaker Andrew Fuller refers to resilience as the ability to bungee jump your way through life. Popular Australian parenting expert Michael Carr-Gregg defines resilience as 'one's ability to bounce back from negative experiences'.[1]

We believe resilience has two very different but equally important focuses: one in the present and one future-focused. Children and young people need to be able to navigate and cope with immediate challenges, frustrations and difficulties, while building up the strengths, skills and psychological hardiness needed to manage future challenges and difficulties. Resilience-promotion is akin to kids spending a portion of their pocket money today, while putting some away for a rainy day. There's an instant pay-off when kids cope with, or succeed in, challenging circumstances but there's also a future pay-off as they've built up some capital to help them manage future challenges.

## The stronger the wind, the stronger the trees

Experiencing life's normal frustrations and challenges contributes to a child's resilience. The seemingly minor disappointments that kids experience – not being picked for a sports team, missing a birthday party due to illness, not achieving marks they expect in a test at school – help prepare kids to manage more significant difficulties such as change, conflict and rejection they may encounter in adolescence and beyond.

Facing up to fears and meeting head-on the situations that cause anxiety rather than avoiding them is not only character-building, but is also the type of behaviour that builds the psychological hardiness that anxious kids need.

In terms of resilience promotion, anxious kids have an advantage over children who breeze through their early years without a care in the world. Anxious kids know what it's like to experience fear, to face a difficult situation with a knot in their gut and their nerves jangling. They also know the exhilaration and relief that comes from conquering their doubts and fears. With tuned-in, sensitive parenting they'll also have the advantage of building a series of skills such as defusion, emotional smarts and mindfulness that will enable them to nimbly navigate future challenges and difficulties whether they be academic, work-related or social.

## Why second-borns are considered more resilient

Second-born kids are considered more resilient than other birth order positions, which is strange when you think that first-borns tend to get all the advantages in terms of attention, resourcing and privileges. The reason for their greater resilience lies partly in the fact that they have to play second fiddle a lot of the time. They are left to their own devices more, so they learn early on not to rely too much on others to get their needs met. There's another reason for their resilience that we often neglect: the innate flexibility that comes with being second cab off the rank. The life of most second-born children revolves around the life of the first-born. The child who comes into the world first sets the agenda for parents. They are the first to walk, talk, go to playgroup, preschool and school. They are the groundbreaker, taking their parents into every new stage of development for the first time. In the meantime, the second child comes along for the ride and learns to fit into the life of their elder sibling. As a toddler the second-born is woken from their nap to pick up the elder sibling from preschool. As a preschooler they may go along to parent–teacher afternoon, or be put into care to free their parents up for the task. As a schoolkid, they are required to watch the elder sibling's first concert or game of sport, and may even spend endless hours watching that sibling train for the game! So most second-borns learn intuitively that they must adapt to the circumstances of others. It's no coincidence that second-borns are most likely to flee the family nest first, either to travel or just to experience living away from home. As adults they are more likely to adapt to new and changing situations. They are also less likely to be anxious or worry about the future, as their attitude to life is far more laissez faire. This flexibility is a huge advantage when it comes to learning to be resilient.

## Getting anxious kids on board the flexibility train

Flexibility is a significant resilience trait we need to nurture in children and teenagers, but doing so in children who are highly anxious is challenging. Uncertainty and lack of control are the drivers of much of the anxiety that many children experience, particularly generalised anxiety. Kids generally become anxious when they are unsure that they can manage a situation. Anxious kids crave certainty and will avoid many situations where they aren't assured of success.

How can parents encourage kids who crave certainty to let go of the need to control every situation and take the risks that come with adaptability? The key lies in providing anxious kids with gradual exposure to situations where they don't feel comfortable or where failure is a possibility. This in many ways is counter-intuitive. As you are aware, anxious kids don't like surprises. They like to feel they are in control and love to know what's going on and what's ahead, which is why social storytelling is so effective. So caring, tuned-in parents will generally spend a lot of time feeding their anxious child the information they need to feel in control. They'll let a young child know at the start of the day which parent is picking them up from school and what they'll be doing after school. They'll talk a child through a new situation such as visiting a friend's house so they know what to expect. They'll talk a child through the first day back at school as thoroughly as they can so they're prepared for the first day. This type of preparation is comforting to an anxious child, but it can also rob them of opportunities to develop the sense of personal resourcefulness that comes from having to 'wing it' themselves without a plan or a script to follow. As much as anxious kids benefit from being provided with a plan to work from, they also need to be placed in situations where there's little preparation or they have to work things out themselves.

## Gradual exposure creates momentum

The legendary figure of Sir John Monash and his groundbreaking approach to guiding his troops to success in World War I provides a surprising insight into how the notion of gradual exposure can be used to change mindsets. Monash, the first

Australian-born general to command Australian troops in the war, refused to sacrifice his troops as cannon fodder in the fields of France, unlike his predecessors. He is widely attributed with turning the tide of the war through his assiduous planning and attention to detail.

Equally pivotal to his success was his ability to change the mindset of the troops from defensive to offensive. This was no mean feat as they'd been stuck in the trenches for months. The troops he inherited in 1918 hadn't experienced military success of any note for more than two years. Monash engineered a series of continuous mini-raids on the enemy so that his troops could be gradually exposed to the feeling of success again. He knew that the more they succeeded in battle, the more his troops would want to experience success. He built a culture of success in his forces by starting small and then harnessing the power of momentum.

This notion of gradual exposure can be aptly applied in families and classrooms to create change, particularly for children who have entrenched habits or fears. Anxious children can be gradually exposed to new or unfamiliar situations without any preparation. We recommend parents occasionally throw away the 'this is what you can expect' script when going somewhere new or different. Let your child experience the discomfort that comes with being unprepared, but also achieve the feeling of satisfaction that comes from knowing they were able to function well despite feeling uncomfortable and anxious.

Anxious kids love to know what's happening each day and can be flummoxed by a change in routine. In fact, many anxious kids feel uncomfortable for some time during the school holidays until they establish a new holiday routine. Don't be afraid to alter their routines occasionally so that they see they can survive having dinner at seven o'clock rather than their usual six o'clock mealtime. This is not about trickery or being deliberately obtuse. Rather, it's artificially creating opportunities for kids to feel a little exposed and uncomfortable and learning that they can function when unpredictability, rather than order, rules. This gradual exposure to unpredictability can help create the momentum needed for anxious kids to become more flexible in their approach and be less fearful of situations that are new, different or previously challenging to them.

## It's all about the group

One thing we rarely read about in the masses of articles and books about the subject is the group-based nature of resilience. While the focus is largely on skilling kids up individually for resilience, it can't be ignored that resilience is a function of groups. If a child belongs to a resilient family, then there's every chance that they'll be resilient too. While resilient parents beget resilient kids, it also must be noted that parents are best placed to promote resilience when their focus is on their family as a whole rather than purely on the child. Child-based parenting, or an approach that puts an individual child ahead of the family, rarely succeeds when difficulties arise. Resilience is best nurtured when the whole family works together sharing the joys, the pain and the challenges of each member. This group-based notion of parenting is problematic in families of two children or less as it's hard not to focus heavily on individuals in small families. When families exceed four children the parenting tends to be more family-focused. Parents are leaders of the gang, delegating a great deal of the work and some of the care to other members. This has the spin-off effect of bringing families closer, and siblings become more supportive of each other when life gets hard. When you have anxious children, work as hard as possible to foster a sense of closeness in your family so that children feel supported and understand that no matter how difficult life can seem, they never have to feel they are facing challenges alone.

# Independence-building makes good parenting sense

Developing independence in children is a no-brainer, isn't it? The aim of parents since the dawn of time has been to raise their children with the express goal of being capable of leaving the nest and fending for themselves. Basically the survival of the species depended on quickly raising the next generation to be autonomous. This goal influenced much parenting practice for many millennia. As life has become easier, families have shrunk and life expectancy has lengthened, and independence-building is no longer the prime parenting objective. It's been replaced by other imperatives, including relationship-building, achievement-orientation and happiness. It's also become harder to promote as the move to smaller families means greater dependence; technology lightens the load, giving kids less opportunity to pull their weight; and urban sprawl makes it harder for kids to spread their wings outside the family home in the same way that kids of previous generations did. This stifling of kids' independence is linked to the increase in their anxiety levels.

# Independence helps lessen anxiety

It would be inaccurate to suggest that no truly autonomous child could become anxious. As we established earlier, there is a genetic connection to anxiety, which can transcend other factors. However, there is no doubt that greater levels of autonomy lead to decreasing levels of anxiety in children and young people in the long run. Independence builds personal capacities in kids. By doing things for themselves they develop mastery over their environment. A child who can tie their own shoelaces is no longer dependent on an adult to do so. A child who is comfortable walking around their neighbourhood negotiating busy streets and roads is no longer dependent on their parents. They

117

are able to visit friends, go to after-school leisure activities and go to the shops on their own. The world suddenly opens up to them, offering a type of freedom that's unavailable when they have to rely on others for transport. These feelings of mastery are important, as they help a child feel a greater sense of control. They are no longer at the beck and call of their parents. But this greater freedom also involves an element of risk. Suddenly the world becomes more unpredictable. Things may go wrong. They may take a wrong turn one day and lose their way. They may encounter people they wouldn't normally meet who make them feel uncomfortable. They may simply experience the extreme elements of wind, rain or heat and have to cope. Each time they successfully deal with situations that lead to uncertainty or fear, they get an important lesson about resilience and build on their feelings of mastery and control.

The experience of fending for themselves is invaluable as it not only builds kids' problem-solving skills and resourcefulness, it also gives them the confidence they need to successfully negotiate future difficulties and, in doing so, overcome their fears.

## How to develop independence

Independence takes many forms but the most important is the development of children's self-help skills. When children are capable of performing tasks safely, let them do so. Maurice Balson, the author of *Becoming Better Parents*, tells parents, 'Never regularly do for kids what kids can do for themselves.' When young children are capable of feeding and dressing themselves, stand back and allow them to do so. When primary school–aged children can make snacks and help prepare a meal, give them the chance to develop those skills. Teenagers who want more autonomy over their lives can be given the chance to create a budget and manage their own expenditure. The confidence gained from this type of self-mastery is immense, and it's easily denied when well-meaning parents and other adults see it as their job to do everything for children and young people. Your job as a parent is to make yourself redundant in a physical sense. You know your job is done when kids aren't reliant on you to do their everyday tasks because they're capable of looking after themselves.

## Give kids responsibility

The next step in independence-building is to give real responsibilities to children and young people. Giving kids responsibility sounds easy, but it can be very difficult to do as it means that we need to let go of the responsibility ourselves. In small families when we know so much about what goes on in our children's lives, it can be very difficult to let go of responsibility. In families of four or more children, it's easier to give a responsibility to kids and then step back to allow them to take real ownership. Due to greater family size, parents tend to broaden their focus and have less personal investment in each child.

## Managing mess-ups and mistakes

The challenge for parents when delegating responsibilities to kids is that inevitably they will make mistakes. Allow a child to pack their own library book for preschool and there will be a good chance that they forget from time to time. Expect your primary school–aged child to remember to pack their own lunch each day and you'll increase the likelihood of it being left at home. Give a teenager the job of taking out the family rubbish each week and there's a possibility that it will be forgotten, meaning the bin will be overflowing the following week. Here's the rub. We need to allow our kids to own their problems and not step in to rescue them. When we rescue kids we take the responsibility away from them. The forgotten library book, the lunch left behind and the overflowing rubbish bin become our responsibilities. Our job is to make it easy for kids to remember their responsibilities and assist them to resolve the problems that they may create through their forgetfulness or simply by making a poor choice, rather than solve the problem for them. When we get very busy it's easier just to sort out the problem ourselves, rather than give kids the space and opportunity to do so themselves.

## Jeremy's story

Ten-year-old Jeremy discovered a great way to earn some extra cash to supplement his pocket money. His family kept chickens, which usually produced far too many eggs for their needs. Jeremy, with his mother's approval, began to sell half a dozen eggs each week to their neighbours. Initially, Jeremy was full of enthusiasm and he regularly dropped them off to his neighbour on the allocated day. He didn't need to be reminded. After a couple of months his enthusiasm began to wane as the entrepreneurial novelty wore off. 'It's Friday. Don't you normally take eggs next door today?' his mother would have to remind him. Jeremy would take in the eggs but begrudgingly, and often in a way that made his mother feel guilty. His mother, feeling underwhelmed by her son's attitude, let him know that the egg business was up to him. She reminded him that the neighbours expected them at the end of the week and if he wanted the money they provided then he needed to remember to do the job himself. After receiving no eggs for three weeks, the neighbour sourced eggs from the super-market and politely let Jeremy know that she couldn't put up with an unreliable supply. Jeremy was flabbergasted.

He thought the neighbour was being unfair. But she wasn't. She was being realistic.

Jeremy received a tough lesson about responsibility. He was learning first-hand that responsibilities may bring rewards but they also come with consequences. When you don't live up to your part of the bargain you fail to experience the rewards. A tough lesson, but that's life.

## The lessons are in the mistakes and stuff-ups

Experiencing these tough lessons that involve disappointment, failure and regret helps develop kids' resilience. Kids learn that they can get over their unpleasant feelings, rather than be debilitated by them. They also learn that although mistakes are awkward and inconvenient, they are not necessarily to be feared. There is in effect little need to become anxious about future events, as failure isn't the end of the world. They will recover. Life will move on. This too shall pass. These are valuable lessons that kids learn when they are allowed to take full responsibility for many aspects of their lives.

## Expanding their horizons

Most adults I speak with look back with misty eyes at their own childhoods, and regret that their children don't enjoy the same freedoms that they relished when growing up. They generally speak fondly of carefree childhoods where they could roam around local streets with relative ease. They reminisce about walking or riding bikes with friends, spending time in parks with a mate or catching public transport to take in a movie or hang around with friends. These were pivotal childhood experiences because they generally took place away from the prying eyes of parents, and sometimes involved an element of risk.

For a child or young person, growing up inevitably means expanding their physical horizons. They move from playing independently at home, to perhaps being allowed to visit immediate neighbours, to then walking around their neighbourhood and beyond. Each step presents small challenges and adjustments that kids (and parents) have to make. Moving around the neighbourhood, for instance, means that children will come into contact with new people; they will go down new streets and visit different parks that will, whether in an urban or rural environment, take them further from the security and safety of home. This greater freedom brings greater unpredictability and more possibilities of adventure for kids. It also means that they may have to draw on their own physical and emotional resources from time to time to get themselves out of sticky situations or deal with uncertainty.

## Encourage emotional self-regulation

The ability to change your mood or regulate your emotions is at the heart of anxiety management. There are many strategies kids can use to alter their mood, including listening to music, playing a game, taking some deep breaths, meditating or doing something physical. Whether it's through relaxation or activity, kids can build up a repertoire of strategies that they can draw on to calm themselves and regain some control when they feel the emotional wheels are taking them to a place they don't want to be.

It's our strong belief that to build our children's capacities to manage anxiety we need to foster the inextricably linked characteristics of independence and resilience in children from a young age. Start by developing a mindset for them by looking for opportunities to promote independence and resilience in small ways. Encourage self-help skills; look for opportunities for children to own their problems; give them some freedom to experience new and unpredictable environments; support them emotionally when things don't go right and help them feel comfortable with fear, doubt and uncertainty.

# 8

# Refining your parenting style

Kids who experience anxiety are helped by two parenting approaches. On the one hand, kids who are worried, fearful or fretting about a future event initially benefit from an empathetic approach. 'I get it' is what they want from an adult so that they feel safe and secure. They also benefit from an adult who says 'I think you can do this', encourages them to face their fears, and also alters the environment to make it a little easier for them to succeed. This kind of parent is usually firmer, though can pose a challenge to any child who wants to avoid the situation or event that causes anxiety. This combination of nurturance and firmness is known as an authoritative parenting style, according to the work of researcher Diane Baumrind who studied parenting styles in the 1960s. A purely nurturant style is known as a permissive style, while a singularly firm style is known as authoritarian.

Neither permissiveness nor authoritarian parenting styles are ultimately successful with anxious kids. All nurturance and no firmness generally means that kids aren't challenged to face difficult situations and so anxiousness continues to spiral. Conversely all firmness and no nurturance and understanding leads to a child or young person feeling unsupported or misunderstood. These feelings are more likely to exacerbate anxiety rather than minimise it. The 'sink or swim' approach advocated by a solely firm style rarely does kids any favours, whether they are prone to anxiousness or not.

When discussing the authoritative approach, we like to use a dog and cat metaphor. Let's begin with dogs. If you have a dog, you'll know it's usually friendly and wants to show love, affection and attention. Dogs are relational and respond warmly to your attention. The 'dog' style of parenting is empathetic, letting kids know that you 'get it' when they are anxious. Cats, on the other hand, are different. They are usually self-sufficient and better able to live quite happily without you. To develop the metaphor, a 'cat' style of parent is more able to challenge kids and encourage them to 'have a go'. They can separate themselves from their kids, step back and not allow emotions to rule decision-making.

Everyone has some cat and dog in them, although most will defer more easily to one style. A parent that is more cat-like in approach is more inclined to push than to nurture. But that doesn't mean they are incapable of applying the dog approach. It just means they need to be a little more conscious of providing the empathy that anxious kids need. Other parents are more comfortable being dog-like, quite unconsciously offering support and understanding when children struggle. These parents, too, can access their cat nature when needed, but this is not their default approach.

## The difference between the cat and dog approaches

The cat–dog styles are expressed through our non-verbal language – our tone of voice, our posture and our heads. A cat speaks in a flat, clipped voice. Their head is very still, their body upright and confident. Cats are calm, quiet and in control. Shouting or aggressiveness is not their style.

Dogs, on the other hand, speak with lots of inflection in their voice, they'll smile a lot and lean in when they speak. It's a warmer, more approachable style. It's the style suited to conversations and building relationships. It's sometimes emotional, is more open and is better used to display empathy.

## Warm cat, firm dog

Which of these two styles do you identify with? If you defer to one then you may have to work a little harder or more consciously to bring the other to the table. In reality, many parents working in partnership with each other will share the dog–cat loads, just as they sometimes play good cop, bad cop when children are less than perfect.

## Don't mix the two approaches up

Get your cat and dog wrong and you'll be ineffective when kids are worried, nervous or anxious. If your first response to a child's anxious moment is to be distant and unapproachable, then you are not meeting your child's immediate emotional needs. Your initial cat-like approach is ill-timed and your child will feel misunderstood and unsupported. Your child needs you to be approachable, or dog-like, when they come to you with genuine concerns. If your child continues to struggle, then the approachable dog needs to step aside and allow the cat to calmly and assuredly prompt the child to take some deep breaths. An excitable or emotional dog will only exacerbate a child's stress when they need to get control of their emotions and thoughts.

Get your response right and you'll be able to give your anxious child or teen exactly what they need. That is, the calmness, confidence and safety that cats provide and the nurturance, validation and understanding that comes naturally to dogs.

## Keep the approaches separate

A common mistake we see is the failure of adults to separate the two approaches. Imagine your son coming home from school very upset. You are not sure what's wrong, but you keep an eye out just the same. The next minute he hurls an insult at his younger sister, causing her to come to you for support. You remonstrate with your son, then sympathetically ask what's troubling him. Most likely you'll get a confused response from your son, as you've mixed management – a cat-like behaviour – with counselling – a dog-like trait. It's best to keep the two approaches separate. In this example, it would be better for you to remonstrate with your son about his behaviour and perhaps send him to his room. Then, when things have calmed down, speak to him quietly about any problems or worries that he may have. This separation will ensure that the firmness of the cat is effective and then gives some time and a different space for the more dog-like approach to work its magic.

## Letting the dog off the lead

When your child is worrying themselves sick and fretting over a future event, such as starting secondary school, it's tempting to be dismissive, particularly if you're not the worrying kind. But this is a time to stop what you're doing, look your child in the eye and really listen to what they have to say. This will help you recognise whether or not they may be anxious. Your child at this point will respond best if their feelings are validated. 'I can see that you're upset. That's understandable,' is the type of response that kids want. You can only truly listen and affirm your child when you let the dog off the lead. A cat-like response won't cut it. Let's take a look at how you can access your inner dog.

The quickest way to access your dog nature is to take a deep breath and speak with your palms facing up. Let's practise this now. Sit or stand up straight, with your elbows at your sides and your hands held out in front of you, palms facing up. Now start a conversation by yourself or with someone else and notice your voice, your posture and any movement of your head. More than likely you'll adopt an approachable style whereby you lean in, your head bobs up and down, and your voice inflects. The upward placement of your palms helps you quickly access the dog side of your nature. Alternatively, imagine you are speaking to a long-lost friend. You'd be leaning in, smiling, making eye contact, your voice would go up and down. You'd even be mirroring your friend's explanatory style as you're getting on like a house on fire. That's the approachable dog at their finest.

## Letting the cat out of the bag

There are many times when the firm parent approach needs to come into play. Stepping back to allow a child to experience the consequences of a poor decision requires some firmness. Insisting a child go to school camp, as you know it's the best decision even though they are anxious, requires nerves of steel from parents. Responding calmly rather than reacting emotionally to a child's anxiety moment takes some effort on the part of a parent. Each of these situations requires parents to be more cat-like – utilising a calm, firm and dependable parenting style. The cat style, when properly communicated, suggests to a child that they will be safe in their endeavours; that they will succeed rather than be flummoxed by a difficult situation.

Want to find your inner cat? Stand or sit up straight, look ahead, keep your head still when you speak, with elbows by your sides, arms out and your palms down. Stay still and you'll communicate in a credible, confident parenting style. You'll also feel more authoritative as you take this cat-like approach. Alternatively, imagine yourself giving a stranger driving directions through a maze of city streets to their hotel. You'd most likely speak using short, clear sentences with a very still and deliberate delivery style. You'd also be watching the stranger's face to make sure they understood your directions. You are processing their reaction all the time. This is the credible cat at their best, spreading confidence through their calm, assured manner.

## Working with your partner

The cat–dog analogy holds true when it comes to partners and their parenting. Often in partnerships the approach each parent adopts will be different. Fathers, for example, are frequently more cat-like when parenting their sons. They often expect a great deal from their boys and are more stand-offish when they struggle with schoolwork, friendships or personal problems. Mothers, when they are attuned to what's happening, will generally use a more dog-like empathetic approach, taking the time to find out what's going on and reassuring their sons that they are in their corner. This type of double-act is effective when a child's emotional needs are being met; when both parents agree with the overall approach that's needed to best raise kids; and when neither openly disagrees with the other in front of the kids.

## Single-parent households – cat *and* dog

Increasingly, children are being raised by a sole parent, whether due to the breakdown of the partnership, or because one parent, often the father, works away from home for long periods, or else lives at home but doesn't participate actively in the parenting process. Sole parents need to be firm cat and nurturant dog all in one package, which is challenging as we tend to default to one style over the other. It helps to be aware of your preference for a cat or a dog approach. This awareness will give you greater flexibility to meet your children's needs in difficult circumstances. There are times when you need to stop and listen to their concerns, and

129

there are times when you need to encourage them to take some risks. You may need to be the comforter, even though that's not your style. Alternatively, you may need to be the firm parent even though you may feel uncomfortable. The cat–dog framework is a practical way for sole parents to offer their children the type of parenting they need to suit different situations.

## A final word on cats and dogs

If you switch unconsciously and automatically between cat and dog, you are naturally charismatic. It's our experience that it's possible to move seamlessly between the two modes but it takes a mix of awareness and practice. If you naturally default to cat mode, then you may have to put some conscious effort into responding with empathy and nurturance when your child is struggling. You may have to remind yourself when your child needs you to stop, lean in, make eye contact and really listen. Alternatively, you may do dog-like behaviours easily but have to work harder to promote independence in your child, or guide your child to take action when they are anxious. In time these switches become automatic as your awareness grows and you adopt new, unfamiliar ways of working with kids.

# Part 4

# Tools for managing anxiety

If you experience anxiety then you'll know that it never really disappears. It's always there in the background. It's a state that needs managing so you can get on with your life doing the things you need to do. There's a big difference between being overwhelmed by anxiety and being able to manage your anxiety and minimise its impact on you and your wellbeing. The former is debilitating both emotionally and physically, causing you to either avoid anxiety-inducing activities or to enter a heightened emotional state in which you micromanage every single activity and prepare for all possible contingencies. You may manage your anxiety but the cost is high, in terms of the emotional energy it takes to get yourself under control as well as predict and manage every variable that may arise. Managing anxiety in this way is exhausting.

Our approach to anxiety is to learn to live with it, rather than fight it. We need to put it to the background while we get on with what we want to do. However, such self-regulation doesn't happen because we will it to. We need a set of versatile skills and tools to call upon in order to manage our emotional and physical states effectively so we don't spin out of control, moving into avoidance or micromanaging modes.

We have identified five tools that are essential for self-regulation of anxiety. We use them extensively ourselves, so we've experienced their impact first-hand. We've also witnessed their positive impact on children and teens. In the following chapters we will introduce you to them so that you can pass them on to your children. Each tool helps to contribute positively to your child's mental health, regardless of whether they experience anxiety or not. However, it's as anxiety management tools that their true value lies. These tools are: checking in, breathing, mindfulness, exercise and defusion. It's time to learn about them.

# 9

# Checking in – an emotional intelligence tool

Can you recall how you woke up this morning? When you first shook your head and cleared the sleep from your eyes, what did you tune in to? Did you think about the day ahead or did you check in to see how you *felt* about the day ahead? Perhaps you did both. It's our experience, backed by the audiences we speak to, that most people begin planning the day ahead when their feet hit the floor each morning. Very few lower their attention to the emotional level to check how they *feel* about the day ahead. Have you woken up nervous or agitated? Have you woken up feeling happy, enthusiastic and motivated? Do you even know?

Anxiety management requires emotional intelligence. In order to manage their anxiety, children need to recognise it. Emotionally intelligent kids are able to recognise a variety of emotions both pleasant and unpleasant. They can also identify less intense emotions such as contentment, calmness and boredom, as well as the more obvious emotions such as anger, fear and enthusiasm that elicit strong behavioural reactions. The next step is to label their feelings; the more nuanced and accurate the better. Then we need to encourage kids to link their emotions to an event, situation or person that may have led to these feelings in the first place. This understanding is a valuable step in the anxiety management process. The skill we recommend to get this emotional intelligence process started is checking in – a simple, powerful skill that kids of all ages from five up can learn and incorporate into their anxiety management toolkit with practice and persistence.

This chapter will teach the skill of checking in so that you can pass it on to your kids. Before we introduce the concept of checking in, we need to establish some basic understandings about emotions.

## Emotions are information

Emotions provide us with valuable information about ourselves and about our children. If you've made an important decision but later changed your mind because 'it didn't feel right', then you've successfully tuned in to your emotions. This 'gut instinct' is information that provides vital clues about all sorts of decisions you may make and directions you may take. For example, when choosing a school for your child, you may have decided on a particular school after weighing up all the pros and cons, only to end up choosing a completely different one because that school 'felt right'. It's astonishing how very rational decisions can be overturned because of a 'funny feeling' we have. In most cases we can verbalise our reasoning quite easily but struggle to identify, or even justify, the source of the emotions that influenced a decision. That's due to the fact that emotions operate in an ever-changing, murky underworld that is foreign to most people. When we're not equipped with the tools to tap into our emotions, we ignore a rich vein of information.

Professor Marc Brackett, director of the Yale Center for Emotional Intelligence and co-creator of RULER, its signature program, says, 'Emotional intelligence needs to become part of the system of a family.' We agree. By making your family a place where emotions matter, you will start to unlock a potentially rich source of information that will not only guide decision-making but help your family be happier, more successful and, importantly, less anxious.

## Emotions are neither good nor bad

There's a tendency to place value judgements on emotions, which is unhelpful. Moods are either good or bad, positive or negative. This black and white depiction of emotions is simplistic and suggests that there are some emotions that shouldn't be experienced. To be human means we feel a whole gamut of emotions every day. Our guess is that during any given day you would have felt annoyance, anger, pride, sadness, worry, disappointment, happiness and joy, just to name a few. It's better to view emotions as either pleasant or unpleasant rather than through the good/bad, positive/negative lens. An emotion such as anger may feel awful but it's not inherently bad or negative. Aggressive behaviour that may stem from anger can be termed bad or negative, due to the adverse impact it can have on others, but the emotion itself is not bad. We, like our children, need to feel comfortable with a range of emotions, and not avoid those that are unpleasant. Anxiety, apprehension, worry, irritation and annoyance are examples of generally unpleasant emotions that your child experiences. It's important that your child is able to recognise and feel comfortable with these emotions, as this is the first step to emotional regulation.

## Feelings and moods are different

The difference between feelings and moods can be summed up quite simply – feelings are fleeting while moods linger. Tune in to your own emotions and you may notice that you feel a number of different emotions. In the one instant you can feel annoyance with

135

a child's interruptions, excited yet anxious about an upcoming job interview and enthusiastic about the night out you have planned with friends in an hour's time. Feelings come and go. Moods stick around and are hard to shift. Moods are feelings that we hang on to because we refuse to let go. A feeling of anger can soon become a big, dark cloud of rage when we keep thinking about an incident, but we have the power to intentionally shift our focus with exercise, humour or turning our thoughts to something else. We recommend that you talk with children and young people about the fleeting notion of feelings so that they can experience them knowing they will soon pass.

## Checking in

It's easy to be tuned in to behaviours and thoughts, but resetting your antennae to pick up emotions – of yourself and others – often takes practice. To this end, the technique of 'checking in' is an excellent emotional intelligence tool.[1] Checking in can be used to identify how you feel at any given moment. The steps are:

1. Stand still and close your eyes.
2. Shut out any external noise and take some deep breaths.
3. Lower your closed eyes below the horizontal plane, to help access the part of the brain where emotions reside.
4. After a short time – less than a minute – open your eyes and acknowledge any feeling you can identify.

This checking-in process should be repeated often through-out the day while you're learning the practice. Keeping a diary of the different feelings you identify and the possible causes for those emotions is a wonderful way to embed the learning of this new tool.

As an adult, checking in should be a regular part of your daily routine. Check in at the start and end of the day, as well as before meetings, presentations and other events that can cause stress or require some positive energy. As a rule of thumb when checking in, try to identify at least one feeling (sometimes there are multiple emotions competing for attention) and then link these to a possible cause. For instance, 'I'm feeling satisfied because I've had a productive day at work', or 'I'm feeling unsettled because I've got some difficult decisions to make', or 'I feel an enormous sense of relief because that project I've been worrying about has just finished'.

## Teaching kids to check in

Checking in is a wonderful tool to introduce to all children and young people, but particularly those who regularly experience anxiety. We don't suggest that kids can control emotions, because both pleasant and unpleasant feelings can come when they least expect them. They can, however, better manage their emotions by identifying how they feel and then reflecting on possible causes. The act of checking in helps children and young people feel more comfortable with unpleasant feelings and builds their capacity to shift their feelings to a preferable or more appropriate state.

Before introducing the checking-in technique to children, familiarise yourself with this important tool. Spend a minimum of two weeks checking in at least three times a day. There is an app developed at the Yale Center for Emotional Intelligence called the Mood Meter that enables you to set timer alerts in your mobile phone. Alternatively, you can use other systems to remind you to check in, or anchor checking in to regular activities such as getting up in the morning, mealtimes or exercise. This anchoring will help you to remember as well as provide fascinating insights into the impact of different activities on your overall wellbeing. Once you feel comfortable with checking in then it's time to introduce it to your children.

It's easier to introduce checking in to your kids if they've seen you do it yourself. This conscious modelling normalises checking in and creates context for your children to practise the skill.

When kids witness you doing it regularly they will begin to see it as normal behaviour that has a positive purpose. Whether it's grabbing a quiet moment in the kitchen, calmly closing your eyes while waiting for a train together, or taking a moment to reflect while watching a sporting event, checking in can be integrated into regular activities. Children and young people will possibly inquire what you are doing. When this happens, explain the process and invite them to join you. Checking in together is a great way to get your child on board.

Avoid pushing it too much if your child resists. However, if possible, explain the benefits, which are: helping them to become more aware of different feelings and able to manage feelings of fear, anxiety and stress when they occur. They will also develop a greater awareness of their emotional world and will be better placed to shift or accept difficult emotions. It will also introduce them to the fleeting nature of feelings and allow them to understand that feelings come and go – including anxious feelings that can make them uncomfortable. Similarly, it will teach them that they can experience multiple emotions at one time.

Teach your kids to use I-statements when they check in. An I-statement identifies a feeling or feelings and links them to a possible event. Examples of I-statements include:

'I feel angry because my friend cheated in a game at recess.'

'I feel unhappy because I've been let down by my best friend.'

'I feel excited because I'm playing in my first tennis final tomorrow but I'm also nervous because I don't want to mess up.'

Encourage kids to say 'I feel angry/unhappy/excited' rather than 'I am angry/unhappy/excited'. The latter is more indicative of mood, which lasts so much longer, while the former indicates a feeling, which is fleeting. The transient nature of feelings is essential to effective management of anxiousness. When we separate the feeling from the person then we're in a position to manage our states. When a person labels themselves as anxious then management becomes so much harder. It suggests that a person has to change if they are to get on top of their anxiety. If we talk about anxious feelings, the inference is that we can manage or change our anxious states when we possess the appropriate tools. The difference in language is minor but the impact is huge.

Help children identify the most appropriate times of the day to check in. Many of the schools that use this emotional-intelligence exercise provide opportunities for students to check in at specific times, such as after recess and lunchtime. First, they set the scene by ensuring students are quiet and calm. They then encourage them to close their eyes, take some big breaths and ask themselves how they feel. When they can identify their feelings – and sometimes there are multiple emotions swimming around inside – they can open their eyes.

Show your child how to prepare to check in. Encourage them to sit or stand still. They should close their eyes and take some deep breaths. Suggest that they tune out from the clutter from their brains by focusing on their breathing. Encourage them to look down at the source of their breathing. Lowering their eyes below the horizon will help them locate the part of their brain where emotions are felt. If they struggle to identify a feeling, encourage them to say any feeling that comes to mind. Often those initial guesses are surprisingly accurate. At first, kids will often say they don't feel anything. If that's the case, push them a little harder to come up with a term. You may even offer some suggestions, such as calm, bored, happy, flat. It's easier to identify extreme emotions such as anger, sadness, exhilaration and fear, but it's harder to identify less intense emotions such as contentment, concern and gratitude.

## Encourage children to keep a diary

Encourage your child to record their I-statements in a diary. This has multiple purposes. First, writing down their feelings helps to build their emotional vocabularies. By naming an emotion a child takes a step towards feeling comfortable with it. The more nuanced their vocabulary becomes, the better equipped they are to shift the way they feel. Labelling is linked to vocabulary development. A child in early primary school will probably possess fewer words in their emotional vocabulary. 'I feel funny inside' may be the limit to their ability to describe their anxiety. A teenager may use terms such as stressed, jittery, troubled and edgy, and over time extend their vocabulary to utilise terms such as overwrought, agitated and perturbed. When you can name it you can tame it.

Secondly, the act of writing encourages reflection. When kids take the time to record their feelings it encourages them to go within and more ably reflect on what they feel. Frequently, a child's initial I-statement can change when it hits their diary, as deeper reflection can give a more accurate depiction of their emotional state. Lastly, a diary provides a wonderful record for a child of their emotional state over a period of time. It also provides evidence of vocabulary development. Anecdotal evidence suggests that diaries can be very motivating, as children see an improvement in their vocabularies as well as seeing patterns emerge in their emotional states.

# 10

# Deep breathing

Ever found yourself on the edge of your seat watching a movie or taking in a close game of sport? If you'd been mindful enough to step back and observe what was happening to you physically, you would have noticed that your posture was taut, your body alert and your eyes open wide. In effect, your body would be replicating the fight-or-flight response as your sympathetic nervous system geared up and prepared you to meet or flee from danger. Your heart rate would have increased and your breathing would have become shallow, preparing you for a quick response if needed. Once the movie had finished or the game ended, after your initial response of relief, joy or disappointment, your body would probably have returned to a more relaxed state. Your shoulders would have dropped, your heartbeat slowed down and your breathing deepened. Situation normal.

However, for many people, children and teenagers included, their normal state is a heightened one. They worry so much about things that are out of their control that their bodies and brains are always on high alert, so they constantly feel stressed and anxious. Usually they breathe from their chests rather than deeply from their diaphragms. If they have a panic attack they'll hyperventilate as their body searches for air. This constant shallow breathing taxes the body and doesn't provide the oxygen they need for optimal functioning. Who would have thought something as basic and simple as breathing was so instrumental in helping us function at optimal levels?

In this chapter we'll look at the place that deep breathing has in both anxiety prevention and anxiety management; how to breathe deeply and effectively; and how you can incorporate deep-breathing exercises into your child's daily life.

## How to breathe deeply

Breathing is essential for our survival. It's automatic. We don't give it any thought until we have breathing difficulties, or we're underwater. Then we appreciate what a life force it is. However, breathing in the right way, at the right moment, is more than merely a survival mechanism. It can help us feel better, prepare better and perform better when we need to be at our best.

You need to breathe into your abdomen, not just your chest. Your body gives clues to the quality of your breathing. Stay still and notice your breathing. If your shoulders rise as you inhale and fall as you exhale, then you are breathing into your chest, known as shallow breathing. If your stomach expands as you inhale and contracts on exhalation, then you're breathing into your diaphragm, also known as deep breathing. In the normal course of the day our breathing patterns will change but most people breathe from their chests, which is both an indication and a cause of stress, pressure and a sedentary lifestyle.

Recognition of the benefits of deep-breathing exercises dates back to ancient Roman and Greek times when doctors recommended the voluntary holding of air in the lungs as a way of cleansing the body of impurities. Deep-breathing exercises include taking big, deep breaths in through your nose, holding them in your diaphragm and exhaling slowly through your mouth. Here's a simple deep-breathing exercise to try:

1. Inhale through your nose and expand your stomach. Count to five while inhaling.
2. Hold and count to three.
3. Exhale fully through your slightly parted mouth and count to five.
4. Repeat for at least two minutes.

Later we'll look at some breathing exercises to introduce to your children, but for now we recommend you practise this simple deep-breathing exercise so you can experience the benefits.

## How deep breathing helps

The physiological benefits attributed to deep breathing are many: it may offer the potential to reduce cardiovascular disease; it encourages full oxygen exchange, which provides the optimum conditions for the body to process toxins; and it allows you to build your endurance for strenuous exercise, as well as improve posture, which in turn may relieve muscle stress.

### Releases stress

If you have a worrier on your hands, then our guess is that you'll be spending a great deal of time helping them forget about their worries. Visiting friends, chilling out on the couch watching a movie, or losing themselves in a digital device are among a range of distractions that many young worriers use. To this list we need to add deep breathing, as it activates the body's relaxation response and so will relieve a person's stress. Deep breathing sends signals to the parasympathetic nervous system of the brain that it's time to relax and rest. As a result the heart rate decreases, the muscles relax, the pupils constrict and the stomach starts to do its important work again. This system takes stressed kids from a frenzied state of worry, even panic, to a more calm state in a short time.

## Calms anxiety

When a child becomes anxious their breathing becomes shallow. In extreme circumstances their breathing is so shallow that they hyperventilate. Taking deep, slow breaths when they become overwhelmed by anxiety is the quickest way to return a child to a calm state. Deep breathing is the only visceral activity that brings the parasympathetic system to the fore. Scientists at Stanford University have identified a small group of neurons that are responsible for calming the brain; these neurons are activated when we breathe deeply. This study gives scientific backing to what we've known for years – that deep breathing calms the mind and relaxes the body.[1]

## Increases energy

Deep breathing increases energy, which is depleted when kids are stressed and anxious. Being on high alert drains kids of the resources they need to be emotionally healthy and to perform at their best. Anxious kids use up more emotional energy than their non-anxious counterparts. Living with anxiety is hard emotional labour. Through regular deep breathing, anxious kids get some of that energy back. When they develop the habit of breathing from their diaphragm, they end up with more energy as their body is provided with more oxygen. With increased energy, kids are better able to think clearly and are more capable of completing the things in life they've put off because they are tired or fatigued.

## Brings kids into the present

Worriers and anxious kids spend a great deal of time thinking about future events. As we have discussed, they often confuse thoughts with facts. At least, their bodies can't tell the difference, and they respond the same way whether a stressor is imagined or real. Just as an imagined tiger can evoke the same type of physical response in a person as a real tiger, so too will worrying about failing an exam. Focusing on their breath forces kids to be present in their bodies, which takes their minds off the events that bring them anxiety and worry.

## Deep breathing is not for everyone

It's worth noting that deep breathing can have adverse effects on a small percentage of people, in that it can increase anxiety rather than decrease it. If you or your child gets light-headed, feels dizzy or becomes increasingly anxious following deep-breathing exercises, then don't do them. Use other techniques such as mindfulness or distraction to calm yourself, or them.

## How to teach deep breathing to kids

Suggesting to a child that you do a breathing exercise together may seem odd at first. You may even be met with resistance. However, don't underestimate your child's willingness to take on new ideas. As a principle, we suggest you explain the benefits in language that kids understand before you introduce anything new or different to their lifestyles. Middle to late primary–aged children and secondary school–aged kids are capable of understanding the impact that breathing has on their physiology and emotions – that it slows their heart rate, relaxes their muscles and helps bring their attention to the present. Assist younger children to understand that deep breathing helps them relax and stay calm. Make deep breathing enjoyable.

A fun addition to your toolkit of breathing exercises is to stand on the opposite side of a table to your child, each with a straw in hand. Take turns trying to blow a small marble from one side of the table to the other, each keeping a slow, steady out-breath.

Consider introducing some breathing games or an activity to relax kids at bedtime or let them join you in a three-minute deep-breathing routine when they wake up each morning. This type of regularity helps to embed deep breathing into their life-style, making it a potent preventative and remedial tool for anxiety, stress and worry.

## Helping kids to practise deep breathing

When anxiety takes hold, the thinking parts of the brain go offline. Breathing mindfully and intentionally helps to calm the amygdala, lessen anxiety and bring the problem-solving and thinking parts of the brain back online. It's a way for anxious kids to show their brain they're safe, so they can then shift their attention to what's important. Dr Chris McCurry has developed some wonderful breathing exercises to introduce to children. We've included three below.

### Finding their breath

It's useful for children to become familiar with the physical sensations that come with deep breathing. It's very comforting to be able to come into the present by conscious use of the breath.

1. Sit with the child. Invite them to breathe naturally through their nose. Help them to find a comfortable rhythm and pace. Their eyes can be open or closed.
2. Ask them to feel the sensation of their breath as it travels in and out of their nose. With each slow inhalation, they can notice how the air they take in is cool against the skin around the edges of their nostrils. Help them to notice how, on the out-breath, the air is warmer, heated by the body.
3. Encourage them to keep breathing and to notice even more subtle variations in the quality of their breath, such as air speed and pressure, temperature, smoothness, any whistling noises, and so on. Invite them to notice the other sensations going on

both inside and outside their body. If they find their minds wandering, teach them to gently bring their attention back to their nostrils and their breathing.

4. Five or ten in–out cycles, done with attention, are sufficient practice for a young child to do at one time.

## Take slow, deep breaths together

A great way to calm an anxious child down is to take some deep breaths together. Here are some instructions you could give:

'Come on, let's take three deep breaths. Okay, ready. Now take a big breath in through your nose. One. Two. Three. Four. Five. Now hold it. One. Two. Three. Okay. Let's breathe out through our mouths. One. Two. Three. Four. Five. Let's do that again.'

It's easier to breathe together with an overwhelmed child or young person if you have both practised together when you are calm.

## Belly breathing

Belly breathing is a great tool for quickly gaining control over the body and steadying the mind when it is alarmed. Belly breathing can be done anywhere, at any time, as it is inconspicuous. You can do it as a form of relaxation while waiting in a super-market queue, to quell nerves before a presentation or to get rid of unwanted tension towards the end of a workday. Here's how kids can practise belly breathing:

1. Suggest they sit in a comfortable chair, with their back straight and feet on the floor.
2. Tell them to locate their belly button with their forefinger, and then place their other hand just above their finger, flat on their abdomen.

3. Then they should breathe in. As they do so, they should imagine that they are blowing up a balloon that's expanding against their hand. They can continue to inflate this balloon with their breath until the inhalation is complete.

4. Next they can breathe out, deflating the balloon until their belly collapses a little underneath their hands.

5. Eight or ten breaths is sufficient practice for one sitting. Practise a couple of times a day – first thing in the morning and at bedtime are usually the best times.

There are many breathing exercises you can do with your kids. We cover many more fun and practical exercises in our online course – Parenting Anxious Kids. You can also find other exercises online. Alternatively, visit your local library or bookstore to locate more resources in this area.

## Making deep breathing part of their lifestyle

If it's to be an effective anxiety management tool, deep breathing should become an integral part of a child's lifestyle. That's not such a big stretch in the twenty-first century. For a start, many schools recognise the educational benefits of good mental health on learning and are now bringing activities that incorporate or promote deep breathing, such as mindfulness and yoga, into regular classroom life. Regular physical activity has now been joined by regular mental health activities as necessary adjuncts to learning in most schools. We suggest that parents capitalise on this normalisation of mental health practices in schools and introduce them as part of their family's regular routines. Just as you might share regular mealtimes together as a way of building a sense of belonging and strong family bonds, we recommend that you spend time together in activities devoted to mindfulness, meditation and deep breathing.

## There's no time like now

So, when do you start teaching your child the art of deep breathing? Developmentally, the ideal time for forming habits in kids is in the primary school years. This is the age when kids adopt many lifetime processes and habits, and although they may deviate from them in adolescence, they'll return to them in adulthood. Habits started under the age of ten, such as sharing meals at the table, developing good sleep practices and exercise routines, become so ingrained that they become part of their way of life.

## Start by practising yourself for ten minutes a day

As with any positive behaviour we want children to adopt, it's always more likely to be successful when parents and other trusted adults, such as teachers, adopt those behaviours as well. Modelling not only normalises behaviours, but serves two broader purposes. As we've already discussed, modelling gives kids permission; in this case, to make deep breathing a fun, acceptable activity to practise. Secondly, they learn the nuances of deep breathing by observing you in action.

Remembering to breathe deeply when under stress can be tricky at first if deep breathing is new to you. We recommend devoting ten minutes a day to deep-breathing exercises. The finding your breath and belly breathing exercises we discuss above will help you to default to deep breathing when under stress. Choose a time of the day that suits you to practise and stick to it. Consider linking deep-breathing practice to another activity, such as a regular visit to the gym or a daily walk or run. By anchoring a new activity to an established activity, you increase the likelihood of developing a new habit.

# Responding to an anxiety moment

Regular deep breathing is a wonderful mental health activity that restores energy, helps kids relax and releases built-up stress and tension. Just as physical activity reduces levels of the body's stress hormones and stimulates the production of endorphins, deep breathing leads your brain to release the body's natural painkillers and mood elevators, and can be a great tool to help a child manage their emotional state when they experience high levels of anxiety. If they are practised in the art of deep breathing, then some simple prompting by a calm yet concerned adult should be enough to encourage them to slow down and breathe. However, such prompting can also have the opposite effect and cause a child to get more upset if deep breathing is new to them. The best course of action in this situation is to invite them to breathe deeply with you. Move close when you breathe together so that the child can match their breathing to yours. This mirroring effect can have a positive impact when a child is panicked or feels that they can't calm down. Naturally, you need to be calm, which has a soothing effect on an upset child. Stay with a child until they have relaxed and calmed down, and their emotional state begins to match yours.

# 11

# Mindfulness

The human mind has a tendency to wander all over the place. You can be comfortably relaxing in a chair when suddenly you recall a past event – a mistake made or an embarrassing moment – and you feel once more the emotion that went with it. Then in an instant your mind can shift to the future, either in anticipation of an exciting event or dreading something new, different or potentially unpleasant. You then experience the emotion that goes with those thoughts – happiness about an eagerly anticipated occasion, or anxiousness about a less-than-pleasant event.

The restless mind has its good and bad points. It can make us feel happy and even motivate us to perform if it gives us a glimpse of a positive future. But it can also drive our insecurity and anxiety if it connects us to events in the past or future that fill us with dread, and make us feel anxious. Our wandering minds need to take a rest and settle into the present, giving us a chance to relax, calm down and focus on what's right in front of us – to be more mindful of the present, rather than the past or future.

In this chapter we'll look at mindfulness as a tool to bring your child's mind into the present moment. We'll look at how mindfulness works, why it's an important skill for an anxious child to learn, and how to bring mindfulness into your own life and that of your family.

## A meditation and a lifestyle

Many readers will be familiar with the practice of mindfulness, as it's been in vogue in the Western world for well over a decade. You may have attended a class on meditation or mindfulness, downloaded an app and practised in your own time, or even been introduced to it by your child, as many schools now incorporate mindfulness practices into classroom life. Mindfulness is a form of meditation that uses the senses as a gateway to bring the attention back to the present moment. It's a way of stopping the restless mind from wandering and grounding it in the present, at least for a short time.

Mindfulness is not just a one-off activity. It's also a way of living that in many respects is alien to us in the current age of mobile phones and multi-tasking. Are you the type of person who, when waiting in a queue, will flick through your mobile phone rather than daydreaming? When you get out of bed each morning, do you give yourself time to wake up fully or do you immediately check your emails? Do you focus on one activity at a time or have you become an expert at cooking a meal, hearing your child read and planning for that important work meeting the next day? If so, welcome to the world of mobile phones and multi-tasking that has become a familiar story for many people. This lifestyle is tiring, stressful and anxiety-inducing, as we're living everywhere but in the present moment. Living a mindful life means that we become more aware of our current surroundings as we focus our attention and our thoughts on one thing at a time. Also, we spend less time on digital devices and more time in the present moment and the sensory world.

# How mindfulness helps anxiety

As we have described, anxiety is an inappropriate activation of the fight-or-flight response in the reptilian part of the brain. That is, our brain is wired to flee or fight when we're in danger. However, our reptilian brain can't distinguish between reality and our imagination. It responds to job interviews, public speaking and dinner parties in much the same way as it would to a real physical danger, if those events fill us with dread and worry.

Mindfulness is a powerful remedy for anxiety as it brings us back to the present, calming our amygdala down, bringing about physical, emotional and behavioural changes. It grounds us in the present moment through our senses, closing down the fight-or-flight response. And it can happen in the blink of an eye. Next time you begin to feel stressed by a future event – when you notice your mind is racing, you feel fidgety, flighty or restless, and emotionally wired or upset – go somewhere quiet, preferably outside. Take some belly breaths, open your eyes wide, look around and call out five sights you can see. If you still feel wired or overly worried, then do it again, and call out three or four sounds you can hear. Continue this process until you feel calm and in control. This simple mindfulness activity won't solve your problems but it will help you feel calmer, more in control and more capable of handling the challenges you anticipate.

Children and teenagers who worry a great deal, ruminate on their problems or overthink them, can easily flick the switch so that their reptilian brain fires off the signals to fight that foe or flee the scene. It's hard to fight or get away when the foe is a thought, spinning around in their head, rather than something tangible and real. Mindfulness can help kids to relax so that they feel less stressed, overwhelmed and out of control.

## The calming presence of an adult

Ever been in the company of an unhappy child and suddenly found yourself unhappy too? There's a reason for this pheno-menon. As social beings we have a tendency to pick up and mirror the predominant emotions of people we are close to. This emotional contagion is a function of groups and it's impacted by two factors. First, we are more likely to pick up the emotions of those we are close to socially, or people we identify with. Second, emotional extremes such as despondency or rage are usually more contagious than more moderate emotions such as annoy-ance or apathy. For instance, a child who catastrophises about the impact of a negative comment made by a peer often finds that a parent or teacher will match their heightened state and will overreact as well.

When kids are upset, emotionally charged or wracked with anxiety they need the adults around them to be calm and in control. If anxiety, a heightened emotional state, is contagious then calm too can be caught, but it takes a little more time and effort as it's a more moderate emotion. Adults who practise mind-fulness are more able to stay present and calm when a child is upset. For a child to become more mindful and grounded in the present, the adults in their life need to be mindful too, and this requires practising mindfulness as an activity.

## This is how you do it

Parents are well positioned to assist kids to manage their anxiety by teaching them critical self-regulation skills. It's essential that we model mindfulness, which is a healthy way of responding to stress and anxiety-inducing situations.

Children see their parents at very close quarters. They witness many of our happiest moments and so see us at our best, and they notice how we approach stressful and challenging situations as well. They see if we avoid challenges or if we take a big breath and tackle them head-on. These are tremendously important lessons for kids to learn. It's the behaviours they witness when adults are under stress that usually have the greatest impact on children. If we blow issues out of all proportion there is every likelihood that children will think catastrophising is an acceptable response mechanism to situations that challenge them. When we respond thoughtfully, calmly and mindfully to a difficult situation, then we show our kids how to respond in similar ways.

## Be present when you are with your children

One of the most difficult tasks of parenting is being present mentally and emotionally with children when we are physically present. We can be in close physical proximity to a child but our minds can be elsewhere, whether pondering a workplace problem, wondering what to cook for dinner or planning an after-school activity. Raising kids means competing priorities, and it's our natural inclination to think, 'What's next?' We know first-hand how difficult it is to be fully present with kids. Life often gets in the way of good intentions, so it helps to have some ground rules to make sure important things happen.

Here are four rules we recommend to rid yourself of multi-tasking and ensure you're present in mind as well as in body when you are at home:

### 1. Ditch the digital devices when you're with your family

It's recommended that parents set rules for children around their digital device use. It's good practice that we follow suit. Develop the habit of placing your digital devices in a designated place in your house, rather than constantly carrying them around with you. This way you'll be less likely to be distracted by unnecessary phone calls, or by getting lost in cyberspace rather than being fully present while you're at home.

## 2. Conduct a mental detox before coming home

The concept of 'The Third Space' created by Dr Adam Fraser is a smart idea that helps you to leave work and other distractions behind when you're with your family. The Third Space is a place you can either physically or mentally go to when transitioning from one activity or place to another. It allows you to momentarily reflect on what you've been doing, relax for a short time and reset your focus on the next activity. Before coming home, stop, reflect on your day, take a few deep breaths to help you relax and prepare yourself to show up and be fully present when you're with your family.

## 3. Do one thing at a time

Multi-tasking, or doing multiple activities at once, is a habit, but it is also a decision that we make. Decide to do one thing, or a maximum of two activities at once and be willing to excuse yourself from other activities, even if it is important to your child. You may be cooking the evening meal, and your child is desperate for your attention. Instinctively, you know that your young person's issue is important and not to be trivialised. Choose one, rather than dividing your attention between two activities. Either set the cooking aside and give your young person your full attention or say, 'I know this is important to you. I want to give you my full attention but now is not the right time. As soon as the meal is prepared we'll sit down together and we can talk.' Prioritise your attention so that you can be fully present and effective in both endeavours rather than doing them simultaneously and not doing either as well as you can.

## 4. Set aside dedicated one-on-one time

We've long been aware of the capacity for one-on-one time to enable parents to build strong relationships with their children. Sharing time and an activity with a child builds your emotional capital, which can withstand the storms and occasional turmoil of adolescence. For one-on-one time to work you need to be fully present with your child, appreciating and feeling comfortable in their company, and enjoying an activity together. This wonderful activity won't necessarily happen unless you set aside some time to make it occur. When children are very young they generally want to spend time with you, so one-on-one time is easy to arrange. As kids move towards adolescence you may have to become insistent and a little creative to catch up, and be present with your kids.

## Introducing mindful practice to children and young people

If mindfulness is to be an effective tool utilised in your child's anxiety management, it needs to be practised regularly. We recommend that you aim for three sessions throughout the day for each child. Mindfulness can be introduced with little explanation to a child from the age of four. When starting out with a young child, practise mindfulness exercises together. Exercises need only last a minute or two with this age group, and involve belly breathing and a focus on their thoughts. Use imagery of clouds passing by or leaves floating along a stream to help young children stand back and observe their thoughts coming and going.

Introducing mindfulness practice to older primary school–aged children and teenagers takes more explanation. Explain how mindfulness brings them into the present using language that they understand. If possible, ascertain their needs so you can relate the benefits of mindfulness to their own lives. For instance, a child may be projecting too much into the future, having difficulty concentrating in class, or continually experiencing worrying thoughts. Explain to kids that mindfulness practice can help them learn better, perform better, and be happier as it helps them live in the present and focus more on what they are doing.

Encourage school-aged kids to practise mindfulness at different times of the day. We recommend that all kids practise a mindfulness activity for four or five minutes before school in the morning as it sets them up to get the most out of a day of learning and socialisation at school. A mindfulness exercise before bed is a great way to help your child relax and get ready for sleep.

## Using mindfulness in an anxious moment

If an upset child is experienced in mindfulness practice, then bringing their attention to the present enables them to self-soothe. You can encourage them to use their senses to bring them into the present: 'Take some big breaths with me. Tell me, what can you see? What can you hear? What can you feel?' Alternatively, get them walking and direct them to focus on their senses, like the feel of the ground under their feet.

If an upset or agitated child is new to mindfulness, then it's very difficult to introduce the practice when their emotions are heightened. However, try to direct their attention towards something that they can see, hear or do. By engaging them in something different you'll be regrounding them in the present moment, and in doing so, calming their amygdala down.

## Mindfulness practices

There are many mindfulness practices that you can try and many resources available. We recommend the Smiling Mind and Headspace apps as they are both produced by nationally recognised, research-based mental health authorities and provide a wide range of mindfulness exercises for children, teenagers and adults. They are also readily available online.

Below are two of our favourite exercises that we have found from experience to be versatile, easy-to-teach and effective to use with a wide range of age groups.

## 5-4-3-2-1 mindfulness

This is a grounding mindfulness practice that is lovely to complete outside where possible.

1. Describe five things you can see.
2. Name four things you can feel (for example, feet on the floor).
3. Name three things you can hear.
4. Name two things you can smell (alternatively, name two scents you love).
5. Describe one thing you're proud of.

## Mindful walking

This practice enables you to combine movement and mindfulness.

1. Stand with a relaxed upright posture and notice the feeling of your feet on the ground. Shift your weight gently from one foot to the other, then share it evenly between both.
2. Relax your arms or gently hold one hand in the other and rest them above your belly button, so their natural swing doesn't distract you.
3. Take a step and feel the swing of your leg starting at the hip; notice each part of the foot as it touches the ground, from your heel, through the mid-foot, onto the ball of the foot and then the toes.
4. Do the same as you take the next and subsequent steps.
5. When your attention wanders, return it to the sensation of your feet making contact with the ground each time. Be kind to

yourself when this happens: each instance is an opportunity to practise returning your attention to your walking. Over time, your mind will wander less, and your attention will return more easily to what's happening in the moment.

6. Maintain a constant pace, a little slower than your typical walking pace.

## Vary the theme

We also encourage you to practise mindfulness with your children in a variety of activities. For instance, you can eat mindfully. That will require them to slow down and really take notice of what they are eating. Encourage them to focus on the taste, the texture and size of their portions. Eating will take a little longer but they may find that they enjoy their food a little more. Encourage them to walk mindfully or go into the garden and take notice of one or more of their senses. Introduce little moments of mindfulness to help them rest and refocus when they move from one activity to another.

## Encourage kids to be kind to themselves

Mindfulness involves bringing kids' attention to the present place and current moment. A child's attitude plays a big part in the effectiveness of mindfulness as an anxiety management tool. If a child stresses or worries about an inability to focus on the present, then they are likely to stop trying to practise. The practice of mindfulness requires an accepting, forgiving, even gentle attitude. Highly anxious kids are generally very hard on themselves, often berating themselves for minute errors that less sensitive kids wouldn't worry about. These anxious kids can become very tense or upset if they can't block out their thoughts when focusing their attention on the present. Help kids to understand that they can't stop thoughts from entering their heads when they practise mindfulness, but they don't have to engage with them. It's important to encourage kids not to be hard on themselves if their thoughts wander. An attitude of self-kindness and acceptance is as much a part of the mindfulness process as the techniques they use to focus their attention on the present.

# 12

# Exercise

Did you spend more of your free time inside or outside as a child? For many parents, the majority of their childhood was spent outside playing some type of game or other. Let's face it, there was less to keep a kid inside than there is nowadays. The TV was a drawcard, but aside from some cartoons and a few favourite shows there was little else to keep us glued to the box. It was also very common for parents to instruct their children to 'go outside and play'. Possibly they instinctively knew that play had mental health benefits, though that thought probably wouldn't have been articulated in the way that most parents could today. Parents simply understood intuitively that a healthy body meant a healthy mind and that children were better off playing outside.

Fast-forward a few decades and lack of exercise or, more accurately, a sedentary lifestyle has raced to the top of the list of public health issues for children. And for good reason, as inactive kids are not only more likely to be overweight but they are also more likely to experience anxiety and other mental health problems. Exercise not only promotes good mental health, it's a tool that kids can use to better manage their emotional states.

In this chapter we'll examine the benefits of exercise to kids' mental health, discuss how we can use exercise and play to

162

manage their moods, and look at ways to introduce exercise to kids who are reluctant.

## Michael's and Jodi's stories

We both have a natural inclination to exercise when we feel down, worried or tense. In fact, exercise is a big part of both our lifestyles. Exercise and sport were also part of our childhood lifestyles. It's no coincidence that the times in our lives when we reduced our exercise were accompanied by poor mental health and a reduction in general wellbeing. We know first-hand that lifestyle factors can sometimes impede our ability to make time to exercise, such as having kids, work and travel. Now, particularly when we feel anxious or stressed, the default position for both of us is to engage in some vigorous exercise that gets the heart rate up and engages the mind. We do so simply because exercise feels good.

## How exercise and movement helps

It's been well established that exercise impacts positively on mental health. The 'healthy body, healthy mind' mantra, which has been around for decades, reflects the long-held belief that exercise and movement is inextricably linked to a person's well-being and positive mental health. The Australian childhood traditionally reflected this view; however, it's now well documented that Australian kids get less exercise than their parents and grandparents, and from both a physical and mental health perspective they are beginning to pay a hefty price, with higher rates of obesity, diabetes, anxiety and depression being suffered by today's children than their predecessors. Before we look at how we can get kids moving more, let's look at how exercise and movement is related to wellbeing and anxiety management.

## Pumps up the endorphins

If you exercise regularly then you may be familiar with the 'runner's high'. It's an apt description of the feeling of euphoria you may feel after completing an energetic gym session, a long run or a game of tennis or squash. This runner's high occurs as a result of your brain's release of endorphins – neurotransmitters that interact with the opiate receptors in the brain to reduce our perception of pain, similar to the way drugs such as morphine and codeine work. Endorphins are known as feel-good chemicals as they reduce feelings of pain and increase feelings of wellbeing. There is also an addictive nature to this release of endorphins, which helps explain why many people get hooked on exercise, even though they may have formerly snubbed their noses at it.

## Creates mindfulness in motion

Just as the act of mindfulness brings a child's attention to the present moment and relaxes the body's fight-or-flight response, an active game or some type of vigorous movement has a similar effect. Our attention becomes highly focused on the game or activity at hand, relieving us of our worries, thoughts and stresses. This is more the case in activities such as ball sports or team events that require greater concentration than repetitive activities, such as walking, in which our minds can wander without affecting performance.

## Relieves muscle tension

When kids are anxious and their fight-or-flight response is on high alert, the heart is pumping blood to their large limbs, preparing them to deal promptly and effectively with the threat. As a result the muscles in their arms, legs and shoulders become tense and ready for action. Once the threat has passed the muscles relax and tension is released. However, when anxiety takes hold the muscle tension lingers far longer than is healthy and the feelings of stress remain. Exercise and movement alongside deep breathing help to relax the muscles and reduce feelings of anxiety that have built up over time.

## Helps us sleep

Exercise can also improve kids' sleep, which is often disrupted by stress, depression and anxiety. We'll discuss in more detail later the importance of sleep for children's mental health and anxiety management. However, for now, it's useful to remember that exercise and movement relaxes the body, relieves tension and helps put kids in the right state for sleep.

## Alleviates anxiety

Anxiety has a way of building up gradually over the course of the day so that at times we're not even aware of its existence. We can come home from work or finish a day of stressful phone conversations and be extremely tense, but not even be aware until someone or something draws our attention to it, such as suddenly snapping for no apparent reason at a family member. It's at these times that physical movement of some type helps.

It's the same with kids. They can bring the stresses of the day home with them, dampening their moods. Alternatively, they may lash out in anger at a sibling or parent as a way of relieving the tension and stress that they feel. Exercise and movement is a healthy way of improving their mood and relieving their stress and tension, whether it's playing a vigorous game with a friend, shooting some basketball hoops on their own or having a run around the park.

## Make exercise part of your family's culture

Parents, as family leaders, are able to make exercise and independence part of the way that 'we do things in this family'. Culture within families is always revealed by children's similarities in values and activities. Not every child will show the same level of interest, or share a trait to the exact same degree, but they will participate and show interest at different levels. The most effective way to introduce exercise and movement so that it becomes a lifestyle, and not just a remedial activity to use from time to time, is to embed exercise in your family culture.

## Get off the couch

If you are a sporty, active type then there is every likelihood that your children will follow suit, particularly if they are in the impressionable preschool and primary school years.

We don't need to go to extreme lengths to get our kids moving, but when parents exercise regularly, play an active sport and set aside time for exercise, they are sending positive messages to their kids about the benefits of movement and exercise.

## Join them

'Come on, let's go outside for a game.'

When was the last time you said this to a child? Hopefully it wasn't that long ago. Children in the preschool and primary school years generally love it when a parent joins them for a game, or for some fun outside. Teenagers will often feign a lack of interest in such an invitation, but many will secretly enjoy the fact that you're willing to join them in a game, even if it's just to prove that they can beat you or they're now fitter or more skilled than you. There are many added benefits to your participation in exercise and movement with your children, including building a strong relationship, encouraging fair play and teaching values such as persistence and honesty. However, from the perspective of encouraging your kids to develop a lifestyle that promotes good mental health and wellbeing, your willingness to regularly get active with your kids is to be applauded. 'Do as I do, not as I say' has a lasting impact on kids.

## Develop a mindset for movement

Improvements in technology make our lives easier and enable us to perform all the activities that our ancestors did, but with less effort. The internet relieves us of the need to visit the library to borrow books for information. The car, soon to be driverless, relieves us of the need to walk. Uber and other home delivery services relieve us of the need to leave the house for an evening meal. Life, if we let it, can take very little physical effort. The alternative, which we highly recommend if physical and mental health are to be priorities, is that we look for and even create opportunities for children to move whenever they can. That may mean encouraging them to walk or ride their bikes around the neighbourhood rather than driving them to or from friends' houses or leisure activities. It may also mean that kids do chores and activities that get them moving, such as helping in the garden, collecting eggs from a family chook pen or emptying rubbish bins. Anything to get kids active.

### Seven ideas to get your kids moving

You may have a child who by habit or inclination spends more time being inactive than you believe is healthy. They may not be the sporty type and prefer to spend their downtime staring at a screen, reading a book or honing their study skills. Despite your best efforts to get them outside and active, they don't match your enthusiasm or effort when it comes to getting their bodies moving. Here are some ideas that are a little different that may just do the trick:

## 1. Count steps on a pedometer

There's no doubt that kids love gadgets, even more so if they measure their own performance. Get a pedometer so they can keep a count of their daily steps. Then create mini-challenges that keep them motivated to move every day. Can you take more steps today than you took yesterday? How quickly can you take 100 steps? How about 1000? What's your record for a week? Maybe you could record some daily steps and create a friendly family competition? The possibilities are endless.

## 2. Thinking outside the playing box

Football, cricket, netball, basketball, athletics, jazz ballet – we're all familiar with these popular activities, but they may not appeal to every child. Let's face it, not everyone is drawn to traditional sports and activities, so consider some alternatives that your child may enjoy, such as rock climbing, dance or martial arts. Be patient, as it takes time for some kids to find the sport or activity that is the right fit.

## 3. Take a break from homework

Insisting kids go outside and play may have the reverse effect and invite resistance instead. 'You want me to go outside to play? We'll see about that' can be the response of some hardliners. Instead, consider suggesting physical activity as a reward, particularly as a break from homework or other school-related tasks. A child may be happy kicking a ball around or shooting some goals if it means they can take a breather from homework.

### 4. Trade 1 for 1, 1 for 2

Some kids love to negotiate with their parents. If this suits your child's style, consider trading time spent on a digital device with time spent exercising, or in activity. What ratio will you negotiate? An hour on a digital device for an hour's exercise and activity? What constitutes activity – is it vigorous exercise or a stroll with the dog around the block? That depends on you, your child and your negotiating skills. Better sharpen up your bargaining powers before you go down this track with your child.

### 5. Look for classes with cool

Not every child is motivated to move, but that doesn't mean you give up on them. Shop around for classes or activities with 'added extras', like those with an inherent 'coolness factor', or that provide an opportunity to make friends, or perhaps have an element of risk or derring-do. Yoga, aikido or skateboarding may just offer some extra cachet to motivate your child to move.

### 6. Perhaps they'd prefer to perform

Some kids like to win, some like to play with their friends and others like to perform. So what is it that motivates your child? If it's the latter then there are many possibilities that combine an element of performance with movement.

Jazz ballet, dance or gymnastics may just be the type of activity that gets your child moving.

### 7. Keep exercise simple

Some kids just aren't into traditional sports and activities. That doesn't mean that they can't become active. Getting kids moving may be as simple as taking the dog for a walk each night, or clambering up a rock wall at the nearest indoor climbing centre. It's the movement that matters when it comes to relieving kids' stresses, regulating their anxious states and taking care of their general wellbeing.

## Getting kids moving in an anxious moment

It can be a tricky proposition to get kids moving as soon as anxiety strikes. When they are overwhelmed by anxious feelings, the most appropriate activity is to engage in deep belly breathing to calm down their amygdala. However, after they've regained composure, try to get them active if possible. You may make an overt suggestion such as, 'Why don't you go outside and have a kick of the football for a while. It'll help you feel better.' Alternatively, you can be a little sneaky and ask them to do a job for you such as take a pet for a walk, or ride a bike to the shops to run an errand for you. At an appropriate age it's important to be open with kids and explain to them that exercise is one of the tools they need to utilise to improve their mood, reduce their anxiety and ultimately get them in the right frame of mind to face those situations that are inducing anxiousness. Invariably, becoming active is the last thing most kids want to do when they are overwhelmed with feelings of dread and worry. Help them broaden their focus away from themselves, and do what's necessary to bring their physiology back to some type of equilibrium. Most kids are fighting their physiology as well as their thoughts when they become anxious, and one of the proven ways of getting them back on track and in control is through exercise, a game or some type of vigorous movement.

# 13

# Defusion

So what are you thinking about at the moment? Do you have the same thoughts now that you did a few minutes ago, or has your mind wandered off in a new direction? It can be hard to notice these things when you are focused on your behaviour, which for most of us means getting through the day, ticking off the to-do list and moving on to the next activity. But tuning in to your thinking is an activity we view as vital to your effectiveness and your well-being, and likewise to that of your children. In this chapter we'll introduce you to the tool of defusion, a tool that will help your child take the power away from their negative thoughts. First, we need to go a little deeper into thought-noticing, a concept we introduced earlier in the book.

## Charlotte's story

Eleven-year-old Charlotte wakes up in the morning and remembers today is the day that she's going on a four-day school camp. She's been dreading this camp because she thinks she'll get homesick and deep down she fears she'll be exposed as the daggy kid no one likes. She's been dogged by these thoughts for months. She's been telling herself, 'I'll miss being away from home' and 'I'm a daggy, boring person.' Whether these thoughts are true or not is irrelevant. They impact negatively on Charlotte's feelings and her behaviour, and they've become her overarching story.

## A thought is not always a fact

Charlotte, like the rest of us, relies on her thoughts to tell her how to live her life – what she should do and what she should avoid. Her thoughts are not always facts, although she reacts as if they are. There are many children who, like Charlotte, can't separate their thoughts from facts, and they suffer because of it. They might avoid situations because they are convinced that they'll fail, they won't be perfect or everyone will laugh at them. Alternatively, they might face up to the situations they dread but the effort and energy it takes to do so will impact significantly on their mental health and wellbeing. Thought-noticing, or metacognition, can help.

## What is thought-noticing?

Thought-noticing refers to the ability to observe your thoughts. In effect, it's thinking about thinking, but not necessarily in an analytical way. It's the ability that we all have to step back and tune in to our thinking.

Children can be trained to practise thought-noticing by tuning in to the continuous chatter and running conversations in their heads. A simple way of introducing thought-noticing is to ask them to stand in front of a mirror and notice what their mind tells them about what they see. They may tell you what they see, describing things such as: 'I've got blonde hair.' 'I'm standing up straight.' 'My eyes are blue.' These are observations rather than thoughts. The difference is slight but significant in terms of the impact on their behaviour and feelings. Challenge them again to tell you what their mind sees. They may make comments such as: 'I'm pretty.' 'I'm so small.' 'I'm no good at sport with this body.' These are thoughts rather than observations, which despite their veracity or otherwise can become the guiding story for a young person. The mind is a great storyteller, so the ability to step back and observe the story is important when it comes to regulating a child's anxiety.

The overarching stories Charlotte is taking to school camp are that she needs her mother and that she isn't popular. The stories show themselves through a myriad of thoughts that come and go. They probably came about as a result of past events, or comments that others made to her. She may have felt homesick on a sleepover a couple of years ago and not been away from home since. She would, therefore, never have tested herself to see if she'd experience homesickness again. She may have experienced some rejection from a group of girls, and their nasty comments still rattle around in her mind. It doesn't matter whether those comments were true and the girls' actions were justifiable or not; what matters is that Charlotte believes them to be true. Charlotte has fused her thoughts together with the facts and they are now the same.

It's important that she's told that she doesn't have to believe these stories or hold on to them. She can choose to see those stories for what they are – thoughts that come and go, that may reflect old, untested beliefs. This is different from the commonly held advice that is often meted out to kids to simply change their negative thoughts to positive ones. Changing a script from 'I'm such an idiot!' to 'I'm intelligent and full of unlimited potential' may sound easy, but this type of reprogramming usually doesn't work. Thoughts, like feelings, come and go and are hard to alter and change. It's far more effective, and realistic, to teach kids to accept their thoughts and give them techniques they can use to distance themselves from those thoughts so they fade and become background noise.

## Sticks and stones

Remember the line 'Sticks and stones may break my bones, but words will never hurt me'? It has been chanted in schoolyards for decades, but it's simply not true. Words can hurt. Nasty words have a way of sticking and hurting long after the person who said them has forgotten them. We can replay them in our heads so often that they seem true. Each time we replay them we repeat the awful feeling of shame, embarrassment or hurt that we first felt. And sometimes the feelings become amplified in the rethinking. Thought-distancing techniques can reduce the impact of words and thoughts on our emotions.

## Distancing kids from their thoughts

Here's an exercise: think of a repetitive thought that upsets or annoys you; that crops up when you least expect it. The thought should begin with 'I am . . .' Some examples are: 'I am arrogant', 'I am hopeless when it comes to sticking at projects', 'I am not good enough'. Hold on to that thought and feel its impact on you.

Now add 'I'm having the thought that' in front of it. Our examples are now: 'I'm having the thought that I am arrogant', 'I'm having the thought that I am hopeless when it comes to sticking at projects', 'I'm having the thought that I am not good enough'. How do you feel about your thought now? Do you feel a little better about it?

This time add 'I notice I'm having the thought that' in front of the thought. So our examples are: 'I notice I'm having the thought that I am arrogant', 'I notice I'm having the thought that

I am hopeless when it comes to sticking at projects', 'I notice I'm having the thought that I am not good enough'. How do you feel now?

Hopefully you noticed that each time you felt that there was a little more distance between you and the thought, its impact was reduced. Adding 'I notice I'm having the thought that' helped give you space and allowed you to step back and notice your thought. This space or distance reduces the likelihood that the thought becomes the story, and is an important technique to teach your child. We don't want to change the words or the story, just notice the thoughts, letting them come and go, reducing their impact.

## Not that old story

Giving their thought a name is another distancing technique to teach kids. If a child constantly thinks they're hopeless, fat or boring then suggest that they name these thoughts accordingly. Suddenly they have the 'hopeless story', the 'fat story', and the 'boring story'. In all likelihood they'll let you know their thoughts as they'll tell you that they're hopeless, fat or boring, so you can help them name the thoughts. Draw their attention to the story they are telling: 'Here's the old "I'm hopeless" story again.' By acknowledging rather than changing it, your child is creating distance from the thought, reducing its impact and the power it can have over them.

There are times when you can challenge a child's self-perception: 'You're not being fair on yourself. You're not hopeless. You are very capable when you want to be.' There are times when children tell us their thoughts so they can feel the reassurance of a loving adult. However, as a distancing technique to reduce the impact that unhelpful thinking can have on kids, naming their story is a terrific self-regulation tool to introduce.

## Sing it again

Beck introduced a fun but effective thought-distancing technique to her daughter when she was fretting over a jazz ballet exam she was taking the next day. Seven-year-old Jasmine told her mother that she kept worrying that she would trip over her own feet during the exam. So Beck started to sing 'Jasmine trips over her feet all the time' to a well-known children's tune ('Bananas in Pyjamas'). Her daughter soon joined her and they both fell about laughing. Beck didn't try to challenge the thought or replace it with a more positive one. By putting the thought to music she helped take the power out of the thought, reducing its impact on her daughter's anxiety.

## Pick a voice

Here's a fun distancing technique that many children enjoy. It asks kids to choose the voices of favourite characters from cartoons, TV programs or movies. They can channel Darth Vader, Shrek or Bugs Bunny as they repeat their negative or troubling thought. Doubtless saying 'I'm too stupid to do well in that test' using a Darth Vader voice will take the sting out of the thought. It certainly helps to reduce the impact of an unhelpful thought on a child's state.

## Is it helpful?

We mentioned at the start of this chapter that the focus should not be on whether children's thoughts about themselves, a situation or event are true, but rather whether the thought is helpful. When Charlotte awoke on the day of school camp and repeated those thoughts she'd been plagued by for months – 'I'll miss being away from home' and 'I'm a daggy, boring person' – she was setting herself up for anxiety. Those thoughts may or may not have been true, but they were certainly not helpful to her at that moment. They were just making her dread what was coming. In actual fact, Charlotte was on the verge of a full-blown panic attack, as she began to hyperventilate. Her mother came to her side and together they practised some belly breathing to calm her down. The fact is, at that point those thoughts were not doing her any favours. It may have helped if she could have verbalised them to her mother, who could then have assisted her to distance herself from the thoughts. However, it would be even better if Charlotte was able to self-regulate. That is, to become aware of her thoughts and use one of the techniques above, or any other defusion technique to enable her to step back from her thoughts and then ask herself, 'Are these thoughts helpful to me now?' If the answer is no, then she should step away from them and begin to face up to what she needed to do – get ready to go to school camp.

## Anxious kids spend a lot of time thinking

Cleverness in kids is usually celebrated by adults with high praise and prizes at school award nights. 'That child is a real thinker' is generally said as a compliment. Yet, often those children who spend a lot of time thinking are also highly anxious. And it's their thinking, or the fact that they spend so much time lost in their thoughts, that can make them highly anxious. They can use their imaginations to think up all sorts of difficulties and challenges that may lie ahead. They can replay those negative thoughts so often that they seem real, and it becomes difficult to separate fact from fiction. Then they worry about what may happen, which can send them into a spiral of anxiety. Rumination left unchecked can be the ruination of a child's mental health. Like a washing machine stuck on spin cycle, their mind goes around and around, chewing over the same thoughts repeatedly.

The ability to step back and observe their own thinking is a positive mental health tool that we need to encourage in kids. We can start by sprinkling thinking starters in our conversations with kids such as, 'What did you notice yourself thinking when you did that?' and 'Is that a thought or a fact?' or 'How is that thinking affecting you?' Asking questions of kids in these ways can get the metacognition process started.

We can also teach kids thought-distancing strategies, some of which we have outlined in this chapter. We can show them how we distance ourselves from our thoughts by thinking aloud. 'I had a horrible thought that I was going to mess up that job interview. I realised it didn't make sense and it wasn't doing me any good so I asked myself, "Is it helpful?" I answered, "No," and then got on with preparing for the interview.' This type of thinking out loud is invaluable to show kids how we approach negative or unhelpful thoughts and prevent them from overwhelming us.

Increasingly, defusion is now tied to resilience as it enables children to approach previously stressful or fearful situations rationally and purposefully. It doesn't necessarily make tackling a situation easier but thought-distancing enables kids to meet a variety of experiences and behave in ways that will help them do what is important to them, rather than avoid them.

# Part 5

# Lifestyle factors that reduce anxiety

Anxiety is complex. Its roots lie deep inside a child's biology, but physiology, psychology and immediate environment also influence how anxiety plays out in a child's life. A child who is predisposed to experiencing anxiousness will benefit from being in a family that recognises their anxiety. If parents ensure routines and structure are in place to prevent unnecessary stress, as well as provide the child with tools such as breathing, thought-noticing and mindfulness, it will help them manage anxious moments. A child's lifestyle also impacts massively on their anxiety. Anxiety management will never be totally effective until it's supported by a lifestyle that promotes a healthy mind and body.

In this section of the book we'll explore seven lifestyle factors that significantly contribute to a child's mental health and well-being. Each of these factors in its own way decreases the likelihood of a child experiencing anxiety, as well as immunises a child from experiencing overwhelming anxiety. When all seven are followed they have a powerful impact on the likelihood of a child experiencing anxiety and their ability to function when anxiety and stress hit. These seven factors are:

- sleep
- nutrition and gut health
- play and movement
- green time
- knowing your values
- volunteering
- healthy relationships.

Let's take a closer look at the lifestyle factors that promote mental health and wellbeing and maximise your child's ability to manage their stress and anxiety.

# 14

# Get plenty of sleep

Living in the twenty-first century presents plenty of barriers to a healthy lifestyle. For instance, the popularity of the mobile phone among young people over the last decade has been accompanied by a decline in the amount of sleep they get. The digital devices that allow a young person to roam through cyberspace are as addictive as cocaine and bring similar arousal side effects. The blue light emitted from mobile phones stimulates the brain, potentially keeping kids awake well into the night. Lack of sleep robs children of their capacity to manage their thinking, exacerbates catastrophising and diminishes their coping mechanisms.

It's well documented that Australia is a sleep-deprived nation. According to a recent study by the Sleep Health Foundation, between 33 and 45 per cent of Australians don't get sufficient sleep, which in turn impacts on their productivity and overall health and wellbeing.[1] That's a staggering figure that shows lack of sleep is occurring at epidemic proportions, but its harmful effects on health haven't received the same attention as binge drinking, tobacco and illegal drug use.

Sleep deprivation is a common phenomenon in many parts of the developed world, including the United States, United Kingdom and Europe. A recent study of the sleep habits of citizens of thirteen countries (excluding Australia) found that 37 per cent of inhabitants of the United Kingdom weren't getting enough sleep, followed closely by the Republic of Ireland, Canada and the United States.

Lack of sleep is not confined to adults. Children share adult propensities to burn the candle at both ends and get by with less than optimum amounts of sleep. Most national health authorities recommend that adolescents get between eight and ten hours a night, yet recent figures show most Australian teens fall well short of that recommended range. According to the 'Teenagers and sleep' page on the Victorian government's Better Health Channel website, most teenagers get between 6.5 and 7.5 hours of sleep per night, which is well below the optimal figure. Anecdotal evidence suggests that the sleep of preschool and primary school children also falls short of the recommended ten to thirteen hours and nine to ten hours respectively.

## Anxiety and lack of sleep

The benefits of good sleep patterns are immense and far-reaching. Sleep impacts kids' learning, their memory and their emotional stability. Positive sleep patterns have also been linked to weight loss, longevity and prosocial behaviours. Sleep helps us function at our best. Conversely, sleep deprivation is akin to functioning in a fog – you may get through the day but you won't be operating at full capacity. And lack of sleep is strongly linked to anxiety and depression. To understand the reasons, we need to take a quick look at how sleep benefits us on a day-to-day basis.

Sleep plays a restorative role. It enables the brain to clean out the toxins it has gathered during a day of energy expenditure, to help create the conditions for optimum learning and thinking the next day. Sleep also rejuvenates the body, repairing tissues and muscles, and allows hormone levels that have been elevated during the day to return to normal. Conversely, lack of sleep impacts on our ability to recover and repair, so it's harder each day to deal with difficult and stressful situations. Consequently, sleep-deprived people experience greater anxiety doing routine tasks and have a higher propensity for pessimistic thinking, which is associated with anxiety.

A lack of sleep disrupts the body's ability to produce serotonin, the feel-good hormone, which helps regulate mood and wellbeing. When the body doesn't produce sufficient serotonin, we use dopamine as a substitute to boost our mood. We get a dopamine hit when using social media or drinking alcohol, which are not healthy activities. These dopamine highs, like fast food, may satisfy us in the short term, but soon leave us hungry for more as there's little long-term lasting or nutritional value. It's little wonder that sleep-deprived people report greater levels of anxiety when they approach mundane tasks.

## Making sleep a priority

The lifestyles of many children get in the way of sleep. Often families fit sleep around school, leisure and family activities, such as mealtimes, rather than regulating activities to ensure kids get the optimum amount of sleep each night. It's vital for parents and teachers to make sleep a major priority for kids. That may mean modifications to the amount of homework kids receive, adjustments to kids' after-school commitments, and changes to family mealtimes so that kids have sufficient time to practise the good sleep hygiene habits necessary for a solid night's sleep. It starts by giving sleep the respect it deserves.

## Optimum sleep framework

Anxiety can often prevent children and teens from falling asleep and this tendency can become a vicious circle. One way to break this worry–wakeful–worry cycle is to develop good sleep promotion habits that utilise a child's natural sleep clock, which is so often ignored at the expense of competing priorities. The following five strategies will give your child or young person the best possible chance to get the sleep that they need.

## 1. Find an optimal bedtime

Traditional wisdom suggests that routine is the key to ensuring children enjoy a good night's sleep. Regularity is just as important for the establishment of good sleep patterns, which are determined by melatonin secretion. Melatonin is the sleep hormone that sets the body's circadian rhythm, the 24-hour sleep clock that helps control when kids fall asleep and when they wake up. Melatonin reacts to sunlight and will adjust according to normal seasonal changes. It loves regularity and reacts poorly to big variations such as crossing time zones or sleeping in for half a day on a weekend to make up for lost sleep during the week. Many of the benefits a child gains from sleep will stem from establishing regularity based on optimal, or perfect, bedtimes that suit them and their lifestyle.

Here's how to find your child's optimal bedtime:

Work backwards from when they need to get up. If they have to wake at 7 a.m. to get ready for the day, then work from this time and add the number of hours recommended for their age group. It's recommended a primary school child should have between nine and eleven hours of sleep a night. Subtract ten hours (it may be nine, eleven or more hours depending on your child's age and sleep history). So 9 p.m. is bedtime. Establish a pre-sleep routine that ensures your child is in bed by 9 p.m. Either provide your child with an alarm or get them up at 7 a.m. If they wake about ten minutes before get-up time then they've found their optimum bedtime. If you have to wake them, set their bedtime back by fifteen minutes. If after three days you still have to wake them, set their sleep time back fifteen more minutes and repeat the process until they begin to wake up before 7 a.m. That final bedtime will be your child's optimal bedtime.

Recommended amount of sleep

| Age | Hours per night |
| --- | --- |
| 3–5 years | 11–13 hours |
| 6–9 years | 10–11 hours |
| 10–18 years | 8–10 hours |

Source: Raisingchildren.net.au

## 2. Create a regular, relaxing bedtime routine

The art of sleep is like the art of seduction – it takes time, requires attention and is all about creating the right mood. Start a bedtime routine at least forty-five minutes out from bedtime; shorter for preschool kids. The aim of the routine is to relax your child, shut down their brain and signal to their body that sleep is near. For good sleep preparation it's imperative to remove mobile phones and other digital devices at least forty-five minutes out from bedtime. If your child has trouble relaxing or switching off consider using calming music, mindfulness, meditation, colouring exercises or some other activity that will help them relax and stop them ruminating. Regular activities such as cleaning teeth at bedtime, having a bedside chat with a parent and reading or sharing a book in bed helps kids get ready for sleep.

## 3. Eat and exercise at the right time

Sleep is easiest when the body is relaxed and the nervous system is calm, so schedule exercise and active movement before meal-times, and schedule mealtimes three hours before bedtime. Food triggers the nervous system, making it harder for kids to fall asleep. You may have to make some compromises, particularly with young children if they go to bed before 7.30 p.m. A 4.30 p.m. mealtime is probably impractical, so just put the biggest gap practical between a child's bedtime and their mealtime.

Exercise, play and movement during the day help children

sleep. Exercise and movement tires kids out, making it easier for them to fall asleep. However, exercise close to bedtime can have the opposite effect, hyping kids up at a time when they should be winding down.

## 4. Create a sleep sanctuary

Kids' bedrooms have many uses. They are frequently used as sin bins, work stations and play spaces. Restrict bedrooms to sleep and relaxation quarters and find other places in the house for time out and reflection, schoolwork and active play. Association is a powerful concept. If kids constantly do homework on their beds then they'll in all likelihood associate bed with work, and may well experience difficulty falling asleep. If there are no other work spaces available, at least encourage them to work at a desk, rather than on their bed.

A child's bedroom should be cave-like – that is, dark, cool and free of electronic devices. Darkness encourages melatonin, which regulates sleep–wake patterns. Remove all electronic devices – melatonin reacts to the smallest of lights, signalling to the body that it should be awake, so digital devices are a no-go during sleep time.

Make sure your child has a comfortable bed and that the air in the bedroom is fresh and smells pleasant. These conditions contribute to a deep, restorative sleep. Keep a moderate room temperature – not too hot or too cold. The body's capacity to regulate heat is reduced when it's asleep, so helping kids choose the right room temperature can help them fall asleep and prevent them from waking up.

## 5. Get up at a regular time

When your child has discovered their optimal bedtime, encourage them to stick to that same time each day. As tempting as it is, particularly for teenagers, urge them to resist sleeping in on weekends, as that will reset their sleep clocks, which will make it harder to wake up during the school week. Kids of all ages usually go to bed later on weekends, but when sleep is a priority, weekend bedtimes should closely resemble the weekday. For optimal sleep, bed and wake-up times need to be as regular as possible.

A good night's sleep has the capacity to lift kids' moods, enhancing their ability to deal with their problems and worries. It's very easy to allow teenagers, in particular, to build a large sleep debt as they go to bed later and later. But sleep debt has serious ramifications, leading to higher levels of anxiety, depression and general distress relative to those who get adequate sleep. Unfortunately, a young person can't go into sleep credit and store up sleep for a busy week ahead. Sleep doesn't work that way. Regularity and routine are the agents of sleep, and adhering to them takes discipline and commitment to making sleep a high priority.

# 15

# Eat well

The 'healthy body, healthy mind' mantra is one that we grew up with. Physical education was a feature of school curricula and parents across the Western world commanded their children to 'turn off that TV and go outside and play'. Physical education and movement were seen as essential for optimum learning and health.

In the current climate where children's mental health is under the spotlight, the 'healthy body, healthy mind' mantra needs some updating. 'A healthy gut, healthy brain' is a more appropriate mantra in an age when we need to focus firmly on kids' mental health before considering their learning capabilities. A healthy gut, or digestive system, equates to a fully functioning brain able to manage the heavy workload required for living in a fast-paced, technological world. So closely are the brain and body linked, the gut is commonly referred to by scientists and medical experts as our 'second brain'.

## The links between gut health and mental health

Scientists are beginning to report on what is known as the gut–brain axis, where early stage/animal studies have found associations between microbiome profiles and clinical mood disorders, such as generalised anxiety disorder. The health of billions of bacteria in the gut is dependent on diet and lifestyle. Typically, kids experiencing an 'anxiety moment' will have high levels of adrenaline (which keeps the brain on high alert), and low levels of GABA – gamma-Aminobutyric acid (which has a calming effect on the brain). These imbalances create conditions in the brain whereby a child or teenager is more likely to experience generalised anxiety and fear, living in a constant state of worry and nervousness. These kids might not be able to relax among friends and family. Some might experience anxiety and fear in a few specific situations, such as when they're surrounded by strangers or when they're high up in a tall building. For these children even slightly stressful situations can bring on headaches, insomnia and muscle tension.

## How the gut works and impacts on anxiety

Our gut microbiome is made up of billions of bacteria that act as a defence against intruders in the gut such as viruses and moulds. They keep the system clean, enabling the nerve cells to produce serotonin and other neurotransmitters such as GABA that help regulate our brains. Serotonin, the feel-good hormone that regulates the ability to stay calm, has the biggest impact on mental health. Around 90 to 95 per cent of the serotonin needed for optimum mental health functioning is produced by nerve cells in the gut. A gut that's full of good bacteria will produce sufficient serotonin to enable the brain to operate efficiently, and is understood to facilitate the biochemical signalling that takes place along the gut–brain axis.

The gut requires good bacteria to keep it healthy. Our diet directly impacts the production of bacteria, and in turn impacts on our mental health and ability to manage stress. Foods that promote good gut health are protein rich (including eggs, oats, meat, cheese), complex carbohydrates (such as multigrain bread) and free from additives and preservatives. They work by stimulating activity in the digestive system and growth of good bacteria in the intestine.

## How excess sugar causes anxiety

There's been a strong anti-sugar movement over the last decade that's seen many books and documentaries highlight the negative effect that excess sugar has on our health, particularly related to increased rates of obesity and type 2 diabetes. Sugar is a common additive in a huge proportion of processed and packaged foods, as well as commercially produced soft drinks. People on sugar-free diets generally report how hard it is to find commercially produced food and drinks that don't contain added sugar. As a result, anecdotal evidence suggests that the best way to eradicate excess sugar from your diet is to steer clear of processed and packaged foods and drinks, eating unprocessed or real foods such as fruit, vegetables and grains.

Sugar in soft drinks or processed food is absorbed very quickly into the bloodstream. This quick absorption causes an initial high or surge of energy. Most parents will be familiar with the notion of a sugar high, experienced when a hyped-up child returns from a birthday party after gorging on sugar-filled cakes, soft drinks and hundreds and thousands. They can't sit still and the noise levels are through the roof. Once the sugar high passes, they will probably be tired, whiny and either annoying behaviourally, or ultra-clingy. Then they inevitably crash.

So what's with the sugar highs? The body reacts to the ingestion of lots of sugar by overproducing insulin as a way to regulate blood sugar levels, then 90–120 minutes later, all that insulin can bring on hypoglycaemia, a state that causes the body to release stress hormones, which may explain your kids' greater levels of anxiety and tension a while after hitting sugary party foods.

Hypoglycaemia triggers the adrenal glands to pump out adrenaline, which keeps the whole system on high alert and leads to a highly anxious, agitated state. What's more, diets high in sugar typically disturb the important work of the gut from producing serotonin, GABA and other hormones necessary for healthy brain function.

You may recall times in your life when you existed solely on sugar, caffeine and adrenaline for periods while cramming for exams, doing late-nighters at work or just when stuck in party mode. You may have functioned for short periods in this mode but when you abuse your body in this way for long enough, you'll inevitably crash – experiencing burnout, a breakdown or some physical ailment that will cause you to stop and change your ways.

## Poor nutrition is entrenched in many kids' lifestyle

It's ironic that in a time when there is such an abundance of food, Western nations such as Australia, the United States and the United Kingdom are reporting high levels of obesity and mental health problems across all age groups, including children. While mental health problems are complex and need to be approached in holistic ways, research suggests that the consumption of food with poor nutritional value is a contributing factor to our current anxiety and mental health problems.

It's clear that good nutrition and eating habits assist kids with anxiety disorders and are an important preventative measure over the long term. The following framework for healthy eating will help keep your kids' bodies and brains in optimal condition for effective performance and good mental health.

## A framework for healthy eating

### 1. Eat real food

The twentieth century has seen a major shift in dietary habits worldwide with a marked increase in the consumption of sugars, snack foods, manufactured foods, take-away foods and high-energy foods. At the same time, the consumption of nutrient-rich and fibre-dense foods has diminished. A peek inside your refrigerator or pantry will reveal how you fit on this scale. If all you can see is jars, cans and labelled boxes and bottles, then your family probably eats a high proportion of processed food. If your shelves are filled with homemade food and liquid, then full marks, as it would seem your family's diet is based on fresh, unprocessed foods.

Choose real foods and minimise your family's consumption of processed, manufactured and pre-packaged and fast foods. Not only are these foods of dubious nutritional value, many also contain high levels of sugar, the enemy of good mental health, as well as other additives that can inhibit the brain's ability to deal with stress. We recommend that you choose foods that are high in complex carbohydrates, which increase the production of serotonin, the mood-lifting hormone that also calms the brain. When choosing carbohydrates, choose wholegrains, such as whole-wheat bread and brown rice, rather than processed choices such as sweets, white bread and white rice. Wholegrains take longer to break down in the body, releasing sugar slowly as the body requires it. Processed carbohydrates give an initial rush of energy, followed by a rapid drop in sugar levels, leaving the body feeling lethargic and, in turn, urging the body to crave more sugar.

### 2. Consume small, regular, balanced meals

The body is its own ecosystem. With proper rest and nourishment it will produce what it needs to function at an optimum level. When you sleep, the brain is in cleaning mode clearing away toxins gathered during a day of energy expenditure. The right nutrition feeds the good bacteria in the gut, keeping the body healthy and influencing serotonin production to shape your mood, and build your coping capacities. This ecosystem relies on good nutrition and thrives on regularity. Provide your children with small, frequent meals that include some protein such as meat, protein balls, cheese or yoghurt and healthy fats such as avocado or nuts that cause a lower rise in blood sugar, preventing sugar highs. Keep snack times regular to minimise mindless snacking and prevent kids from overeating sugary treats.

Kids will often use food as a self-medication when they feel anxious or to get their minds off their worries. In some cases it can lead to binge eating. The reliance on food as a comforter when under stress quickly becomes a habit that's hard to break.

## 3. Start the day with protein and complex carbs

Children who experience anxiety are generally keenly sensitive to any physiological changes in their bodies. Having a dip in their blood sugar levels can feel similar to a panic attack. A breakfast high in protein and containing complex carbohydrates will help keep your child's sugar levels steady throughout the day. To get protein into a child's morning diet, turn back the clock thirty years to when it was common to give them a breakfast that included eggs, oats and milk or natural yoghurt. Eggs are high in protein, easy to serve and contain choline, a nutrient that curbs anxiety and boosts memory. Serve an egg up with some wholegrain bread or toast and you're ensuring a gradual and sustained blood sugar release throughout the morning. Skip the high sugar breakfast cereals and try oats served with natural yoghurt. Add a glass of milk, and you're providing the nutrients that the gut needs to do its work.

## 4. Drink plenty of water

You probably know that dehydration is commonly linked to dry lips and feelings of thirst, but did you know that it's also linked to anxiety? Dehydration sends the body into panic mode, with the heart racing, leaving a person feeling light-headed and agitated. The line between adequate hydration and dehydration is a fine one. Very active kids can often forget to drink water and become dehydrated. They can also become so engrossed in a task such as studying, playing a video game or watching a TV program that they forget to hydrate. Encourage children to keep a drink bottle on hand at all times and to drink regularly. They should resist the habit of drinking sweet drinks when they are thirsty so they don't binge on sugar. Water as the go-to for regular hydration should become a lifelong habit for kids.

## 5. Keep kids away from caffeine

It's been well established that caffeine either in the form of coffee or energy drinks impacts negatively on sleep. Caffeine is a stimulant that fires up the fight-or-flight response, making it a bad option for those with a predisposition towards anxiety. Excess caffeine alone can trigger an anxiety attack. People with an inclination towards anxiety can experience nervousness, restlessness and fear after drinking just one cup of medium-strength coffee. Doctors commonly recommend that adults with anxiety disorders or symptoms limit their caffeine intake.

Caffeine intake, while formerly largely an adult concern, now needs to be addressed in kids. While children in primary school years may not be coffee drinkers, caffeinated energy drinks and soft drinks are becoming popular with this age group. Teenagers are often imbibers of energy drinks. However, as a child's brain is developing, it's advisable to completely eliminate caffeine from their diet until they reach at least fifteen years of age. This means keeping caffeinated products out of the refrigerator and substituting energy drinks and coffee with healthier choices such as water or a banana smoothie.

Good nutrition is the foundation of good mental health. Just as a house needs to be built on a firm foundation to make it resistant to changing weather conditions, good nutrition is the building block for optimal physical and mental health. Parents are raising kids at a time when fast food, processed food and sugary drinks are widely available, and frequently placed on high rotation in media and advertising campaigns. However, parents are in the prime position to influence their children's eating choices. It starts by choosing wisely the food you add to the family larder and extends to the conversations you have about healthy eating, and modelling moderate consumption and consistent eating habits yourself. Healthy eating is a lifestyle, not something you only do when you're sick or want to lose weight.

# 16

# Go play

Speak to most adults about their happiest childhood memories and inevitably they'll talk about play. Some will recall games such as hide-and-seek or tag, riding around the neighbourhood on a bike or playing organised sports and games. Others remember their involvement in creative activities such as building forts, putting on plays or playing dress-ups. In most cases their parents were largely ignorant of what they were doing.

So what's the definition of play? A quick online search brings up terms like 'enjoyment and recreation', 'spending time doing enjoyable things' and 'taking part in a game or entertaining activity'.

Borrowing from the work of Dr Stuart Brown and Dr Brené Brown, we define play as involvement in an activity that is fun, free and involves flow.[1] It's an activity that's highly anticipated (fun), self-directed (free) and that we don't want to stop (flow).

## The 3Fs of play

Fun – the game or activity needs to be enjoyable, engaging and active rather than passive

Free – it is freely chosen and self-directed rather than an activity that the participant is encouraged, or expected to do

Flow – participants get lost in time and don't want the activity to end

## The decline of play

It's been widely reported that the amount of time kids spend involved in play has declined over the last few decades. Children are increasingly involved in adult-initiated activities that are purpose-driven and highly scheduled. Soccer, violin lessons, jazz ballet classes, after-school tutoring, anyone?

When was the last time you heard someone say: 'My daughter is going to play this weekend'? We hear parents talk about how weekends and after-school hours are taken up with driving kids to various sports, activities and lessons. It's not that anyone has set out to eliminate free play, but we just don't value it as highly as we do purposeful, educational, organised activity.

### Michael's story

Recently, I took my five-year-old granddaughter Astrid to a playground that contained some challenging play equipment. Astrid loves testing herself physically on climbing equipment, but she is the type of child who looks before she leaps. She definitely erred on the side of caution when she approached a challenging part of the playground. It was a scary three-metre thrill ride on a ring that slid from one platform to another, with a drop of half a metre. She held on tight and squeezed her eyes shut, before taking a big breath and a leap of faith, jumping off the platform. She didn't open her eyes until she arrived at the other end. Jubilation replaced the look of uncertainty on her face.

Immediately she went back for another ride, and another, and another.

Children face many such challenges when they are able to play freely in outdoor environments. These challenges encourage them to face up to their fears, cope with uncertainty and feel comfortable with unpleasant emotions.

## Locus of control

Fear is a central emotion behind most forms of anxiety. This fear is born from a perceived lack of control, which can drive kids to obsessive preparation and perfectionism or cause them to avoid situations where success is not assured or that cause them discomfort. Play is essential to raising resilient kids because it helps them build the competence and confidence they need to positively shape their environment. Importantly, it helps them build the sense that they have power over their own lives and are able to influence and change events that worry them. The opposite, a sense of helplessness, is associated with anxiety and depression.

In their book *The Danish Way of Parenting*, the authors Jessica Joelle Alexander and Iben Dissing Sandahl lament the parenting shift in developed countries to a style that promotes an external locus of control whereby children are encouraged to be more motivated by adult ambitions than their own interests and goals. They write that 'younger and younger children are feeling a lack of control over their lives. They are feeling this sense of helplessness earlier and earlier. This rise in external locus of control over the years has a linear correlation with the rise in depression and anxiety in our society.'[2] With the increase of pressure being exerted on kids to perform at their best, the need for play has never been greater.

## Play is therapeutic

In Chapter 12 we discussed how movement and exercise relieves stress by releasing endorphins, feel-good chemicals that enhance mood and wellbeing. Exercise and physical activity is one of the tools that kids can use to alter their mood and help them better manage their anxiousness. Play that keeps kids active helps fight anxiousness. It helps kids feel good and is therapeutic by nature. Play researcher Brian Sutton-Smith pointed to the negative impact of the lack of play when he wrote, 'The opposite of play is not a present reality or work. It is depression.'[3] Experts know that people who experience depression almost always have eliminated fun and play from their lives. Sadly, it's not just adults who have jettisoned play; many children have had their free play replaced, or at least squeezed out, by organised activities that now take up the greater part of their time.

## Getting more play in kids' lives

The term 'child's play' is problematic and emblematic of our attitude to play. If a job is determined to be child's play it suggests that the job is easy, taking little or no effort or skill to perform. The term is demeaning to children and dismissive of the place of play. Play is essential to maintaining a person's happiness and positive wellbeing.

Play is serious business – it's nothing to be flippant about. It takes some effort for us to write this as we are both highly driven to succeed, and frequently feel uncomfortable when we're not writing a blog, cooking a meal or doing something productive. You want us to play? We've got too much to do for such a frivolous activity. But play – doing things because they are enjoyable and not just to achieve a goal – is essential for healthy human development. It seems odd to suggest that kids, those traditional kings and queens of play, should play more. But they should, as they don't do it enough. And play shouldn't be discarded in adulthood. We hope that play and playfulness will accompany your child into adulthood. What follows are five ideas to encourage a lifestyle that includes play.

## 1. Give kids permission to play

Researcher Brené Brown claims that busyness is one of the main impediments to people's happiness in Western countries like the United States, the United Kingdom and Australia. The current cultural norm is that if you're not busy then you must be failing, or you don't have any drive. In a world where fifty-hour-plus working weeks are acceptable, we frequently don't allow ourselves time or give ourselves the permission to play. If adults don't play, then kids aren't likely to follow suit. We need to give kids permission to play and be frivolous, and incorporate some play in our own adult lives.

## 2. Allow time and space for play

In many cases it's not that we devalue play, it's just that it falls to the bottom of our priority list. For most kids play now comes after school, homework, chores and adult-initiated activities are completed. Kids, like their parents, are busy. Lack of time is the enemy of play. We do urge you, particularly if you have a child who is stressed or experiencing anxiety, to look at their schedule and set aside some downtime so they can play.

The type of play that's beneficial for kids in terms of mental health promotion and safe risk-taking generally occurs outdoors. When kids move away from the four walls of home, the world becomes a little more uncertain, even unpredictable. Whether it's in the bush, a park, a safe street or a well-designed playground, when a child is play-fighting with a friend, swinging from a branch or simply jumping off some rocks, it helps to remember that they are not only learning how to manipulate their environment, they're learning how much stress they can endure.

## 3. Give kids the freedom to play unobserved

A great deal of play that's valuable for kids goes unobserved by adults. Child-initiated activities such as building a cubby, arguing with a friend over the rules of a game or going for a nonstop tennis ball-bouncing world record don't have to be witnessed by an adult. Enjoyment is the aim. They need no adult judgement or comment except, 'I love that you play.'

Resist the urge to hover when kids play and also to know everything that's going on in their lives. Kids need the freedom to play without well-meaning adults jumping in to protect them from harm, make suggestions or even stop them from facing their fears. Letting go of control is anathema for many parents, but in the interests of encouraging children to play we suggest that you give them some space.

## 4. Encourage lone play

Play has many social benefits for kids, including learning how to negotiate with someone bigger, smarter or more needy than you; knowing what winning and losing feels like; and experiencing rejection and other social difficulties that playing with friends and siblings brings. Boys, in particular, often compete with each other for the title of the fastest, longest or fiercest, which helps develop their confidence and coping skills.

Solitary play has enormous benefits too. Time alone allows kids to reflect and process what's happened to them during the day. Resist the temptation to keep kids' days filled with activities and friends. Encouraging alone time, whether it's doodling, hitting a tennis ball against a wall or completing a jigsaw puzzle, allows a child the chance to unwind and process the day. In the modern nonstop world it can be hard sometimes for a child to find time to be alone. But it's important that they do.

## 5. Get other adults involved

Worried about other parents judging you poorly if you let your child off the leash and adopt some of these kinds of play principles? We're pretty quick to judge each other these days. In 2009 Lenore Skenazy, journalist and champion of the Free-Range Kids parenting movement, won the monicker of America's Worst Mom when she wrote a column for *The New York Times* explaining how she allowed her upper-primary-school-aged son to ride the subway unsupervised. Skenazy has led a crusade ever since being the subject of a public backlash, urging parents and teachers to give kids the freedom they need to take sensible risks that will lead to their independence. As Skenazy famously found, when you give kids permission to play, explore and problem-solve, in all likelihood you'll open yourself up to criticism.

On the other hand, you can involve other adults in a movement that allows kids to play. Be prepared to explain that your child is taking a break from organised sport because they need some time to themselves. Create discussion with other parents about the value of free play for kids' healthy development and mental health. Be an advocate for the benefits of play, both for your child's mental health and for your own wellbeing.

We may look back wistfully on our own childhoods, but our memory is selective. Recollections of being hurt, experiencing conflict and disappointment or the frustration of having nothing to do are forgotten, while great memories of fun and enjoyment are amplified.

It's our contention that the good far outweighs the bad, and that we'd be doing kids a huge favour if we encouraged them to go outside and play.

## You can be playful too

Have you ever jumped out at your kids to give them a fright? While it might seem counterintuitive, this kind of playful behaviour can help protect kids against anxiety.[4] Called challenging parenting behaviours (CPBs), they include behaviour such as playful wrestling, rough-and-tumble play, encouraging assertiveness and risk-taking, and teasing (as long as it's not taken too far). Fathers are more likely than mothers to play with their kids in these ways, but when either mothers or fathers incorporate CPBs into playtime, their kids are less likely to be anxious.

Kids love this quality time with one or both parents. It's fun, relaxing and creates an opportunity for kids to express themselves physically while experiencing safe risks. From each CPB interaction they're either led or they venture out of their comfort zone, experience some anxiety and learn that they're actually okay. They learn that the world isn't such a scary place after all.

Challenging parenting behaviours give kids opportunities to learn that they're resilient and capable, and that anxiety-provoking situations are manageable.

# 17

# Enjoy green time

In 1981 futurist Faith Popcorn coined the term 'cocooning' to describe the trend of people staying inside their homes rather than going out for entertainment. She predicted that the rise of the VCR, home delivery of fast food and the home services industry would keep people cocooned in their homes. This was a bold prediction at the time, but even Popcorn couldn't have foreseen just how big an impact technology was going to have on people's lives. New communication, education and entertainment technologies developed since the turn of the century have accelerated the cocooning effect in multiple ways.

Families can now meet most of their daily needs without taking a step out the front door. For most, the family dwelling is a very comfortable place – too comfortable for children to leave. They don't need to leave home to play with a friend. They can hook up online, even play a game together. The lure of the outdoors has faded. Australian kids are now indoor kids. And this aversion to outdoor activity is not just an Australian phenomenon. A recent UK study found that children spend half the time playing outside that their parents did.[1] British children now spend four hours a week playing outside compared to the 8.2 hours that their parents used to. Studies in the United States and other parts of the Western world show similar results.

## Technology is the headline act

Digital technology is the crowd-puller when it comes to children. Children are bombarded with new entertainment mediums, from more established technology like TV and film to cutting-edge games, social media and mobile phones. There are more diversions than ever to occupy the minds and time of children. Information technology is widely used at school, so the amount of time children spend in front of a digital screen is ever-expanding. Until recent years the impact of technology use on kids' lifestyles and mental health hasn't been widely considered. The NSW Education Department recently became the first state in Australia to initiate a study into the impact of technology use on children and teenagers with the aim of providing recommendations for its safe use by students at school and at home.

## The opportunity cost of screen time

Spending time outdoors has traditionally been linked to exercise and sport, which have positive impacts on health and character development. Most of us intuitively know that the time spent outside, particularly in nature, is good for our overall well-being, but there's now a mountain of evidence linking time spent outdoors with positive mental health outcomes for kids. Time spent in front of the artificial blue light of screens robs kids of time that should and could be spent outdoors.

It's simplistic to say outdoor activities are universally good, indoor activities are bad. However, the shift towards a more sedentary childhood spent largely indoors has gone too far and needs to be redressed as part of an overall strategy to reduce anxiety and stress levels and improve mental health in the long term.

## It's all about green-time

There's a wonderful worldwide movement encouraging people to spend more time in the natural environment. Perhaps the most extreme and most interesting example is forest bathing, or *shinrin-yoku*, that began in Japan in the 1980s. The idea of *shinrin-yoku* is simple. It refers to quiet, sedentary time spent in a natural environment where people can metaphorically 'bathe' in the forest and experience nature using their senses of sight, hearing, smell, taste and touch. When people spend time in a forest, or a green environment, they feel calmer, less stressed and more relaxed. Anyone who has spent time in a forest or bush setting will have automatically felt this. Anecdotal accounts of the rejuvenating benefits of time spent in the forest or bush are now backed by solid evidence showing significant health improvements, leading to long-term reductions in anxiety and depression.

A recently released, large-scale study from the United Kingdom reveals the extent of the benefits of green time on community health. Researchers from the University of East Anglia drew on a mass of data from 143 studies, involving 290 million participants from twenty countries. The team correlated time spent in green spaces with over 100 positive health outcomes, including reduced risk of heart disease, type 2 diabetes and lower blood pressure. The mental health benefits of time spent in green space were significant. The researchers found a direct correlation between time spent in the natural environment and a lowering of mental health disorders such as anxiety and depression. In particular, spending time in natural environments reduces cortisol levels, the stress hormone that helps maintain our anxious states.[2]

Other studies point to the positive impact of green time on kids' anxiety levels when combined with exercise. Young people sleep better, relax better and feel better when they're active in green environments. The human brain was designed to cope with outdoor living, so it feels most comfortable in that environment.

Millions of years of evolution can't be overturned in a few decades. There's a familiarity to spending time in forests or the bush. Spending time in green spaces is like meeting a long-lost friend, where we instantly feel at home in their company.

## Getting more green time in kids' lives

'Turn that screen off and get some exercise!' That would work . . . once or twice. Realistically, digital devices are here to stay. We don't want to turn back the clock and remove all electronic devices from kids' hands. The benefits are overwhelmingly positive when used well, but kids' technology use needs to be managed, or at least monitored by parents and teachers. It's not always possible for a child to go to the bush or find some green space for a mental pick-me-up when they're feeling down. We need to make sure kids manage their screen time responsibly and get the green time they need for optimum mental health.

## Help kids manage screen time

There are three ways to approach kids' digital screen time. One way is to throw your hands in the air and put the management of their digital device use in the too-hard basket, then let them do as they please. Do this and you risk raising a self-centred child (because they spend all their time glued to a device), as well as placing them in a dangerous position to be exploited by strangers, leaving them defenceless against cyberbullies and letting them learn for themselves the pitfalls of posting pics and selfies online. That's without considering the impact that continuous mobile phone use may have on your child's mood and wellbeing.

Another way to approach digital screen time is to place a full or partial ban on technology use at home. Not only would this put you at war with your child, but it gives you little or no influence over how they can safely and smartly use digital technology.

The third, and preferred, option is to take an active part in helping children make the best and safest possible use of digital technology. That means sitting down with your kids and working through some basic ground rules. Start with what Martine Oglethorpe, aka The Modern Parent, calls 'no brainer' rules. Martine notes that although rules often change when it comes to technology as kids get older, parents should still make some universal rules for the whole family. 'It may be that there are no phones in the bedroom at night. It may be that there is no technology after a certain time of the day. It should certainly be that devices never ever come to the table at dinner time.'[3]

Once some family rules are devised, Oglethorpe advises parents to take into consideration the impact that time on devices is having on other aspects of their lives. She says parents need to consider how their children are coping with their digital use. If technology use causes them stress, fatigue or anxiety, the amount of time they spend on digital devices and specific usage should be addressed. Similarly, if they don't have time for other activities such as homework, hobbies and family meals, then they may need assistance or coaching to better manage their usage. We applaud Oglethorpe's approach of encouraging parents to be involved with kids' digital usage using a mix of modelling, monitoring, friendly discussion and boundaries to help ensure that kids' mental health is not at risk and that there is ample time for other areas of life, including spending time outdoors.

## Expose kids to nature

You don't have to sell the family home and head bush if you want your kids to experience the benefits of green time. Urban dwellers need not despair. The East Anglia meta-study found that time spent in urban green spaces such as parks and green street spaces had a similar calming impact with the same mental health benefits as time spent under a lush forest canopy. You don't have to wait until weekends or holidays to give your kids a healthy dose of green time. Urban dwellers, and that's most Australians, can look much closer to home. Beaches, parks, backyards and urban walking and bike trails can provide the green space needed to promote good mental health.

## Take the indoors outside

Kids can do a lot of things outside that they currently do inside. They can meet friends after school at a park, playground or soccer field rather than at home. Birthday parties and other gatherings can take place at the beach, a park or in the bush. Outdoor play dates for young children can be arranged at parks, creeks or lakes. Make the outdoors your new normal for kids' and family activities rather than continually defaulting to indoors.

## Do as the Scandinavians do

Scandinavians have a penchant for indoor plants, which makes perfect sense. They experience long, dark, cold winters, which keep them inside for long stretches. Recognising the positive effect of greenery on mood and wellbeing, they fill their homes and apartments with plants and shrubs. Researchers aren't sure how greenery works on our brains. One theory is that we respond positively to things that are good for us and we associate protection, nutrition and survival with trees and forests.

Take the Scandinavians' lead and place some greenery in your home, kids' play spaces and bedrooms. Involve kids in their selection, their maintenance and choosing suitable locations at home.

## Go play in a forest

How about a family holiday with a difference? Rather than taking your family to a theme park, head bush for some solitude,

211

adventure and fun. Spending time in the bush is a green prescription for kids who lack everyday access to green spaces and the measurable health benefits they provide.

Time spent in nature almost always makes you feel better. It's time that's rarely wasted. Yet it's time that's increasingly being denied to kids due to their busy lifestyle demands, increasing urbanisation and the modern penchant for cocooning. In the same way Americans living on the east coast in the 1800s were encouraged to 'go west', in these anxious times let's make 'go bush' the modern mantra. More green time is a wonderful natural remedy for anxiousness and a natural antidote to many of the ills caused by increased screen time.

# 18

# Know what matters

## Avoid patterns of avoidance

For many children, avoidance of anxiety-inducing events becomes a pattern of behaviour that initially serves them well. In the short term, feelings of stress, worry and anxiety are removed. But many kids who practise avoidance experience doubt, guilt and in extreme cases self-loathing, as they can't escape feelings of disappointment for taking the easy way out.

Avoidance can take many forms, including procrastination, self-deprecation ('I'm not good enough'), oppositional behaviour and lack of interest. Avoidance becomes a vicious cycle where the more kids stay away from challenging events or social situations, the more anxious they feel when similar situations occur. Exposure to anxiety-inducing events is the key to helping kids overcome their anxieties rather than allowing anxiety to dictate their lives.

## Evan's story

Nine-year-old Evan was invited to a slumber party by a school friend. He was thrilled, because Evan loved nothing better than hanging out with his mates and having fun. It didn't take long for his enthusiasm to be replaced by a feeling of dread. Evan had been diagnosed with obsessive-compulsive disorder, which meant he rigidly stuck to his daily rituals. He had developed many rituals at school such as lining up his pens on his table to start the day, laying his lunch out carefully on the lid of his lunchbox before eating, and always coming and leaving by the same school gate. His mates knew he had some strange habits but they were unaware of the extent of his obsessive behaviours, as he'd managed to keep most of them hidden. However, his OCD showed itself fully at home through his ritualisation of many routine tasks such as eating his meals, preparing for school and getting ready to go to bed. He knew that bedtime rituals would be thrown out the window at his friend's slumber party.

Evan worried about the slumber party for days. He pictured himself getting ready for bed at 8.10 p.m., which was the exact time he began getting ready for bed each night. Cleaning his teeth came next. He saw himself unscrewing the cap and placing it open side up on the bathroom sink. He began cleaning his teeth from the back left-hand side of his mouth, working his way around his lower teeth until he reached the other side where he turned the toothbrush to the front of his teeth and methodically worked his way around to the left-hand side of his mouth again. He repeated the process on his upper teeth. The same order as always. Then he went to his bedroom and lay his pyjamas out on his bed. His bedtime ritual went on like this until his light went out at 8.30 p.m. He felt comforted by his routine. He knew it helped him sleep and he feared what would happen if he altered it.

He confided in his mum that going to the slumber party was way too hard. He expected his mother to agree, as she had allowed him to miss the school sports day earlier that year because just thinking about it made him want to throw up. His mother surprised him. 'I get that you're uptight about going to Jake's party and I think I know why, but you know how much you like having fun with your friends, and Jake is a special mate. I think you should go. Let's figure out a way that you can go and have some fun without feeling so anxious about it,' she said to him. His mother folded her arms in a way that indicated that no more discussion would be entered into.

Evan's constant ruminations about the slumber party fed his anxiety. In return, avoidance became his main goal. He thought that he'd be fine as long as he stayed away from the slumber party. His mother intervened by reminding him about how friendships and having fun were important to him, and that his anxiety shouldn't prevent him from attending. His mother was insisting that Evan be guided by his values rather than his anxiety. Evan's mum should be applauded because although she was taking what may seem a hard line, she knew it would help her son in the long run.

Evan's mother helped him map out a more flexible bed-time ritual that left out some of the more minute details but kept enough to help him feel comfortable. She encouraged him to practise the new bedtime ritual a number of nights before the slumber party. She also alerted Jake's mother, who agreed to keep the other boys busy around bedtime, providing Evan with the privacy he was used to.

215

When the time for the party came, Evan was nervous, but he was determined to join in. Comforted by the fact that he had a practised plan, he was able to relax and enjoy himself. His bedtime plan went off without a hitch and Evan was left wondering what all the fuss had been about.

## Helping kids to be guided by values

Traditionally, values were viewed as being akin to a moral compass, whereby qualities such as honesty, discipline and respect were to be taught and developed in children. But this narrow interpretation is not entirely useful if you are an anxious type of person. We believe values are the personal principles and deeply held interests that guide our behaviour. Dr Russ Harris, author of *The Happiness Trap*, says of values:

A value is a direction we desire to keep moving in, an ongoing process that never reaches an end. For example, the desire to be a loving and caring parent is a value. It's ongoing for the rest of your life. The moment you stop being loving and caring, you are no longer living by that value.[1]

Values are important because they help us behave in ways that really matter. Everything worthwhile takes effort: raising kids, building a business, learning the guitar, winning or performing well at sport. These activities are challenging. It's easy to give in before achieving success. But that's where values come in. When we know what's really important, we'll pay the price in terms of effort, whether physical or psychological, to overcome any challenges we meet. As Harris succinctly puts it, 'Values provide a powerful antidote, a way to give your life purpose, meaning, and passion.'[2]

In Evan's case, having friends and fun are core values as evidenced by his previous behaviours. He loves having friends over to his place and he always seems to be surrounded by mates of different ages at school. Evan is often laughing and playing around with his younger siblings. His values are evident in his interests and the way he behaves.

Directing anxious kids to take values-driven action is a core pillar of our approach to helping children manage their anxiety, rather than being debilitated by it. In previous chapters we've outlined many strategies, such as practice and gradual exposure, that parents and teachers can use to help kids take the action required to achieve their goals. But it's essential to help kids understand what's important to them. The following ideas will help you and the kids in your life gain a greater understanding of their values, why they are important and, significantly, how to put those values into action.

## Know what's important

There are many values-clarification activities that you can complete with primary-aged children.[3] Here's an example of a values-clarification you can use with upper primary and secondary school children:

'What would you do?'

Encourage a child or teen to write answers to these questions:

1. If you had billions of dollars to spend however you wanted, what would you buy and what would you do?
2. Okay, so now you've got everything you've ever wanted, what would you do next? Would you do something creative? Help other people? Start a business? Take action about a cause you believe in? Make a list of at least ten things you'd do if you had everything you wanted.

This list will give you and your child an insight into what's really important to them.

Another way to gain an understanding of kids' values is to help them tap into their interests and passions. Look at how they go about their interests and the qualities that they display. If a child loves building cubbies outside or making up plays, then it may be that creativity matters a great deal to them. A teenager who contributes to social service causes, coaches younger children's basketball in their free time and is helpful at home may have service and generosity to others as core values. A child who consistently works through every task, paying massive attention to detail, may value excellence and high performance.

Here's another simple way to help you understand a child's values. Finish this sentence with an activity:

My child is happiest when _____

Some examples:

My child is happiest when they are playing outside on their bike.

My child is happiest when they are helping the underdog or have a cause to fight for.

My child is happiest when they are playing music of any sort.

In each of these examples it may be that we have to look a little deeper than the obvious answer. A value displayed by playing outside on a bike could be a love of the outdoors or a love of adventure. A child who constantly supports the underdog and loves a cause to fight for may value compassion or social justice. The child who is happiest playing music could value creativity, performing or relaxation. Tapping into what kids love to do will help give you an understanding of the values that give their lives real meaning.

## Connect kids to their values

Develop the habit of connecting kids to their values. One way to do this is to paint a picture of their values during general conversations. Comments such as: 'One thing I've noticed about you is that you seem to be at your happiest when you're challenging yourself in some way. It's amazing how you always seem up for a challenge.' Or: 'You seem to love beautiful things, whether it's a sunset, a picture or even a pair of shoes.' Or: 'I love the way you ask so many questions. You can also get lost in a book. Could it be that you are curious?'

Connecting kids to their values, or what gives them joy, has a powerful effect as kids crave this sort of self-knowledge. When they can recognise what drives them they are more likely to challenge themselves socially or in other areas, despite any feelings of anxiety.

## Colin's story

Colin should have been a sports champion. As a child he was a star at every sport he tried – football, cricket, tennis. You name it, he could play it. He was naturally gifted so he didn't have to work hard to perform well as a kid. In his mid-teens he had the luxury of having professional teams in football and cricket coaxing him to join them. He chose football and went into the AFL draft. He was taken high in the draft but he only lasted four years in the AFL system before leaving the game for good. When he reached a professional standard, he came up against players of lesser talent who had worked hard and made the sacrifices needed to succeed when they were younger. They were prepared to do the work needed to succeed at a professional level. Colin had never had to work hard at his sport, and wasn't prepared to do whatever it took to succeed. He was a victim of his precocious talent.

There are many stories in sport like Colin's in which people aren't willing to put in the work needed to succeed. This willingness to do what's needed is relevant in all walks of life, and is especially relevant for kids who experience anxiety.

## Two sides of the same coin

Dr Chris McCurry has a great activity he uses in his therapy sessions to help kids rise to the challenge of achieving their aims. He calls it 'two sides of the same coin'. He shows the children a large circle with 'The Good Stuff' written on it. On the reverse are the words 'The Challenging Stuff'. He uses this to remind kids that if they want to achieve good stuff, such as doing well at school, enjoying loving friends, and playing a sport at a high level, then they need to also do the hard work that's needed, give something up or put themselves into situations where they feel uncomfortable or anxious. It's a great reminder that anything worthwhile doesn't come easy. Success and challenge is a package deal.

Knowing what matters is a life quest for most of us. The search for meaning and purpose is a search for happiness and fulfilment. This process can start in childhood. By helping kids understand the values they hold true, as opposed to imposing external values such as respect and honesty onto them, we give them a wonderful tool to approach life. Importantly, we believe that when guided by their values, kids are more likely to take the necessary actions, with support, that will help them achieve in the areas of life that are important to them, despite discomfort and anxiety. The adherence to personal values and the continual search for an understanding of those values is part of the lifestyle of an emotionally mature, happy person.

# 19

# Volunteer

There's a worldwide movement towards volunteering and it's easy to see why. Most people who volunteer their time in the service of others report feeling a greater sense of purpose and enjoyment, and an increased sense of belonging and connectedness to others. Studies also reinforce tangible physical and mental health benefits, particularly lowering participant anxiety and depression levels.

Volunteering is frequently associated with retirees and people in the later stages of their working lives. But the reality is quite different. According to the Australian Bureau of Statistics (ABS), the age group of fifteen to seventeen years has the highest volunteering rates, with 42 per cent of that age group involved in voluntary work. The next group, at 30 per cent, is the thirty-five to forty-four age group.[1] There are relatively few statistics that look at the volunteering rates of children under the age of fifteen, but we suspect that the figures may be higher than many people would think. Schools have long promoted social service, and groups such as the Scouts and Girl Guides, as well as sporting clubs, have consistently viewed service as integral to their mission.

## How volunteering helps kids who are anxious

Research on the positive mental health benefits of volunteering for kids is unfolding, but we have some suggestions about why we believe it helps. One theory is that oxytocin, the neurotransmitter that regulates social bonding, increases when young people volunteer, helping them manage their internal stress in social situations. Volunteering then has benefits for children with social phobias who struggle to meet people. In more general terms, volunteering has three positive benefits for kids who are predisposed to experiencing anxiety, which can be summed up by the acronym ICE: impact, connection, empathy.

### Impact

Volunteering has the potential to increase a child's self-efficacy. When a child runs an ill neighbour's errands, coaches a younger age group's netball team or sets up a garage sale to raise money for a food bank, they experience first-hand how their efforts can impact others. Often kids who experience anxiousness worry that they don't have the capacity to handle a new situation or event. They fear that they will fail or make fools of themselves in new or unplanned situations. Volunteering builds their capacity in comparatively low-pressure situations, where the focus is on someone or something else. It allows kids to build their skills in relatively non-stressful situations and, importantly, experience how their efforts can have an impact, no matter how small, on others.

### Connection

Most volunteering involves other people. Whether it's being a ballkid at the tennis, tutoring a child who needs homework help or organising a run-a-thon to raise money for a worthy cause, service for others enables kids to form connections with people outside their normal demographic. It's been well established that social connection to family, school and community is a strong protective factor for young people's mental health. Families and schools generally work very hard to ensure young people feel that they belong; however, their connection to and meaningful engagement in the community can be a struggle to obtain. Volunteering is a great vehicle for developing a young person's engagement in the community, which is purposeful and lasting. And it's a great way to meet friends and forge new relationships, which, as we shall see in the next chapter, are essential for their long-term mental health.

## Empathy

Empathy has a profound impact on how kids live. Without empathy a child has difficulty experiencing respectful relationships. An inability to identify with how someone else is feeling makes it easier for a child to reject, bully or intimidate others. Kids lacking in empathy are also likely to be very self-absorbed and lack a sense of proportion when events don't go to plan. A child who thinks about others, particularly people in comparatively difficult situations, is more likely to keep their own challenges in perspective. Empathy is experienced, rather than taught, through exposure to other people's difficulties. Kids need to relate to a situation or person to develop real empathy. Volunteering helps kids develop empathy as it helps them experience and understand how other people live.

## Putting volunteering in your family frame

How do we encourage kids to take up volunteering and, more significantly, stick at it so that it becomes a part of their lives? Data collected by the ABS shows that in 2014 more than two-thirds of volunteers (70 per cent) had one or more parents involved in voluntary work. Nearly half these people had volunteered for ten years or more. Once parents started volunteering, their children were likely to follow. These are startling figures that reveal not only the power of modelling but the extent to which parent modelling impacts on family culture.

Looking for volunteer opportunities that complement the interests of your child can also help. For instance, if your child is an animal lover, perhaps a local shelter could use a dog walker. If they are sporty, then find a local sports club that could use an extra hand.

## Volunteer with kids

The most effective way to develop a culture of volunteering is by parents working alongside kids in a voluntary capacity. This can be done in many ways, ranging from cleaning up a neighbour's yard together, to working backstage at an amateur theatre, or joining an international voluntary aid project as a family. There are also many community projects, such as Clean Up Australia Day, that offer one-off opportunities for families to become immersed in public service.

## Kids help at home without being paid

A child's early years set the tone for the rest of their life. Austrian psychologist Alfred Adler, the father of the theory of individual psychology, maintained that children's early family experiences determined how they belonged to all the different groups in their life. If their contribution to the family was encouraged and valued, they would more than likely develop the healthy lifestyle view that 'I belong to my family/class/workplace through contribution, therefore I'm a valuable group member'. When children's early attempts at helping and contributing to personal and family well-being are thwarted through lack of opportunity, low expectations and over-protection, then children inevitably find other ways of belonging, including: 'I belong when I can put others in my service', 'I belong when I get my own way' or 'I belong when I'm the smartest/prettiest/most powerful person in the group'. You may recognise some of these people as workmates, friends and partners.

If you want your child to develop a sense of belonging through service, we recommend that they should help regularly at home without being paid. In this way, they are more likely to grow up with a healthy sense of belonging, where they think 'I can help' rather than 'What's in it for me?' We recommend that children receive pocket money but without linking it to chores. The very nature of belonging to a family, just like any group, is that we contribute positively to its ongoing wellbeing. In this way, service and giving becomes a part of life, a pattern that's hard to shake.

# 20

# Build relationships

The well-known adage 'A problem shared is a problem halved' reflects the truism that sharing problems and worries with a supportive friend or family member helps a person feel better, giving them perspective and providing reassurance. There's been a great deal written in recent years about the fracturing of community and the isolation that many people feel. Increasing urbanisation in most developing countries is frequently linked to a weakening sense of community. Long working hours, communication technology and cocooning are some of the other culprits widely identified as weakening community ties.

Conversely, positive family relationships and peer connections have long been associated with good mental health and wellbeing. In the 1980s pioneering resiliency researcher Bonnie Bernard first identified positive social interaction with family and friends as a powerful protective factor for young people. Since then a wide body of research has confirmed the positive impact that family and friends can have on children's wellbeing. They can also have the reverse effect. Family dysfunction and negative peer interactions can be the cause of anxiety and depression in a child.

# What do positive relationships look like?

Children are able to function at their best when they enjoy close interactions with family and friends. We have identified three key characteristics in family and friendship groups that contribute to positive or nurturing relationships that assist children to respond to challenges and problems.

## Positive family relationships

Positive family relationships that enhance good mental health and equip kids to face challenges such as change, social difficulties or traumatic events, are those that are loving, supportive and promote a sense of belonging.

### Love

Bernard's resiliency research found that 'having a warm and affectionate father or mother was significantly associated with an adult's social accomplishments and wellbeing'.[1] In effect, family affection has a long-term positive impact on a child's functioning and wellbeing.

### Support

Supportive relationships exist when parents are non-judgemental, available for kids to confide in and willing to listen when kids have problems.

### A sense of belonging

When kids are valued, any problems they have or needs they express won't diminish their sense of place in their family.

Positive family relationships are best summed up as places where kids feel safe and secure; they can freely practise the necessary skills that they need for successful social living; and know they won't be rejected no matter how poor their behaviour or how difficult life can become.

## Positive peer relationships

Peer relationships and friendships have an important developmental function for children. In early childhood, friends are the first entry point to the wider social world outside their family. In childhood years, friendships help a child form their identity, but their family usually remains their strongest reference point. In adolescence, friendships become the stepping stone for life to adulthood, when they begin their own family. In lieu of starting their own family, friendships become a substitute, fulfilling the need for belonging, acceptance and affection or intimacy for many young people. Every parent will know that their child's friendships can be a dual-edged sword – the cause of both pain and happiness.

Developmentally, some ages are more problematic when it comes to friendships. For instance, early adolescent girls can be less than pleasant to each other, and their friendships often wax and wane from one day to the next. The mental health of girls in this age group will frequently reflect the behaviour and attitudes of their primary peer group. When relationships with friends go well, they feel great. When rejection, ostracism or conflict occurs, they become moody, unhappy and cantankerous at home.

Studies show there are a number of recurring qualities in the positive friendships of young people. These include loyalty, honesty, openness and authenticity. Through our work with children and teenagers over a long period of time we've identified three key characteristics that exist in almost all healthy friendships for young people: encouragement, acceptance and generosity. These qualities work best as a package.

### Encouragement
Good friendships are energising rather than draining. Time spent with a good friend leaves a person feeling better than when they

started. They exude a sense of positivity rather than negativity, which occurs in friendships that are toxic.

### Acceptance

A good friend is accepting of another's differences and is truly interested in their life. A child is more likely to take a friend into their confidence when they are accepting and know that when they reveal their innermost self to that friend, it will not be repeated to others or used as currency in a later dispute.

### Generosity

Positive friends are generous with their time and their spirit. Many children fail at friendships because they won't open themselves up to other children. Generosity takes many forms. It's the generosity of spirit shown when a child is happy for a friend who wins a medal, earns an A+ at school or gets genuine applause at their concert. It's the capacity to make sacrifices to help friends out when they are unhappy. Generosity is shown when a young person is vulnerable enough to confide some of their worries and difficulties with a friend.

## Nurturing positive relationships

There's no magic formula for promoting healthy relationships. One of the basic tasks of parenting is to socialise children so that they can enjoy healthy relationships with people from different backgrounds, and in different situations, including in their immediate family, at school and in the workplace, with friends and peers and with a life partner. From a mental health perspective there are a number of strategies adults can use to ensure kids are strongly connected to their family and also enjoy positive relationships with their peers. Let's explore some key relationship-building strategies.

## Create a strong food culture in your family

Ever noticed how countries with strong traditional food cultures, such as Italy, France and China, pride themselves on the strength of their families? It's no coincidence that countries that truly value food, cook meals with care and flair, and eat at a leisurely pace, also highly value family relationships. The act of sitting down and breaking bread together on a regular basis is probably the most powerful ritual that parents have at their disposal to build a strong family. In strong food cultures, preparation of food is generally a family affair with most members lending a hand at some stage, whether it's buying ingredients, cooking, laying the table, serving or cleaning up after the meal. This involvement creates shared ownership, making mealtime a treasured event rather than a refuelling exercise.

In most strong food cultures, the meal table is the fulcrum around which the family is built. There's an expectation that everyone joins the family at mealtime, rather than allowing kids to eat meals in their bedrooms or in front of a screen. Mealtimes are not to be taken lightly. There's significant evidence to show that there's a correlation between young people's good mental health and those that eat regularly – five to six times per week – with their family. This is no surprise, as mealtimes offer parents and young people the opportunity to talk with each other, which can be therapeutic when they are presented with challenges. Regular mealtimes also offer parents the opportunity to monitor their children for signs of anxiety and depression, which may otherwise go unnoticed.

If mealtimes have never been a huge priority in your family, start by making one meal a week a family affair. Get everyone involved in some aspect of the meal, keep all digital devices away and do your best to make it an enjoyable experience.

## Put vulnerability on display

We often hear the lament: 'I can't get my kids to open up to me.' It's also a challenge we've experienced in our own families. Some children are like open books and willingly share their problems. Others can be conversational clams, refusing to open up.

Kids frequently need the time and space to process their problems before they come to a parent. Many boys, like cave-dwellers, will go to their bedrooms to think things through before discussing their problems with an adult.

Regardless of all your best efforts, sometimes young people just won't open up. There are no guarantees that kids will seek help with their problems and worries. It helps, though, if loving, trusted adults can show them the way. That may mean that parents and teachers display vulnerability and talk to kids about some of their difficulties. Talking about your own anxieties in safe ways not only shows kids how to talk about problems and share their emotions, but it gives them permission to do the same. Fathers, in particular, are well placed to guide their sons to open up on an emotional level, but they need to show them how.

## Discuss friendships openly

Parents frequently worry about the negative impact that the wrong type of peer or friend can have on their child. The term 'peer pressure' alludes to the influence that others may have on a child to behave in ways that are unsafe, illegal or just plain stupid. How much to interfere with a child's friendship choices is a conundrum for many parents. An effective way to influence children to make good friendship choices is to create family conversations about healthy friendships. In particular, it's critical for the sake of a child's mental health to be able to differentiate between a clique and a positive friendship group. Ongoing conversations about positive friendships are helpful and can be peppered with questions such as: 'Is that how a good friend behaves?'; 'What does a good friend look like?'; and: 'Is that how you want a friend to act towards you?' It's useful when discussing the nature of friendships with teenagers to use their values as a reference point. For example, 'Doing well at school is important to you. Does your friend's behaviour help or hinder you in class? If it's the latter, you may need to figure out a way to be their friend and still keep up with your schoolwork.' Conversations that help children delve into the complexity of friendships can help them formulate their own ideas about friendships. They also help them practise the self-reflection needed to explore their own role in their friendship problems and develop the efficacy to be good friends themselves.

## Encourage kids to enjoy wide friendship circles

Mental health experts agree that one sure way for a child to improve their mood over the long term is to build their social connections. Unfortunately, anxiety can prevent a child from making new social connections. If this is the case in your family, we recommend that you assist your child to experience social situations a little at a time until they feel comfortable with a new group. We also urge you to encourage your child to develop a number of different friendship groups inside and outside of school. This will not only provide some social insulation should one friendship group prove difficult, it will also ensure your child meets many different children and forges relationships with children from different backgrounds. Social fluidity – that is, the ability to develop relationships with a broad range of people – is a higher level relationship skill you can nurture in childhood.

A child's relationships with their friends and family contribute enormously to their wellbeing, particularly when managing mental health issues like stress, depression or anxiety. While personal relationships can at times be the cause of significant stress and anxiety to a child, the overall positive effect of healthy relationships on wellbeing far outweighs the negatives. Parents are in an ideal position to help their kids develop the skills and attitudes needed to enjoy healthy relationships in all areas of their lives. It may take some coaching, cajoling and coaxing at times, but the results in terms of long-term mental health outcomes and lower anxiety make it worth the effort.

# Part 6

# Managing significant anxiety issues

The question on the mind of anyone parenting an anxious child is always: 'What can I do to help?' Paradoxically, the short answer is: 'How long have you got?'

On top of the symptoms of anxiety that cause distress in children, parenting an anxious child puts parents on an emotional rollercoaster. Some days are extraordinarily difficult and painful, some days feel perfectly and wonderfully ordinary, and then there's everything in between. We'd trade places with our anxious kids in a heartbeat given the chance; it's hard to see them feeling distressed, harder still if you don't know how to help.

We invite you to look at your situation differently – to see each day as an opportunity. There are daily actions you can encourage that will make a tangible difference to your child's experience of anxiety in the moment and in between anxious moments. Each day is peppered with pockets of time in which you can extend your child's understanding of anxiety, where it comes from and why; as well as guiding them to practise the skills that show their amygdala they're safe, calm their nervous system and restore their thinking brain back into action.

The skills you teach and reinforce through daily practice add to their mental health toolkit, staying with them while they're firmly under your wing and long after they've flown the nest.

Remember, the goal here isn't to rid your child of their anxiety. Attempts to do that can disappoint and actually undermine progress improving their mental health. Everything you'll learn in the following chapters will support you to help your anxious child move their anxiety from centre stage to the wings, maybe even the dressing room or the theatre carpark.

Different types of anxiety disorders respond to different approaches. Breathing and mindfulness are the core skills and strategies at the heart of the management of any type of anxiety that we have explored in previous chapters. Next we want to share with you another layer of understanding that can be applied if your child's anxiety diagnosis is more serious or complex.

You'll learn what to expect when you visit your GP to talk about your child's anxiety, the ins and outs of a mental health care plan, how finding a psychologist is like buying a pair of jeans, and how to explain to your child what a psychologist does and how they can help.

# 21

# When kids need more assistance

Some anxious kids need professional help to manage their anxiety. This help will come from any one or a combination of professionals, including general practitioners, psychologists, counsellors, occupational therapists, exercise physiologists or psychiatrists. The most appropriate health professional for your child will depend on their diagnosis and age.

We stongly recommend making an appointment with your GP as a first step. They're the gateway to other health professionals who provide treatment in the form of therapy and medication or a blend of the two. Medication helps to smooth out the peaks of anxious symptoms for some kids; therapy or counselling provides psychoeducation, understanding and support, and teaches powerful thinking skills.

Some children feel confronted by the idea of seeking professional help. The personal nature of anxiety causes embarrassment for some who will baulk at the idea of sharing their personal information, even with their family doctor.

Your child might be a willing participant in seeking assistance, or might dig their heels in and refuse to cooperate. After our anxiety presentations we're regularly approached by parents who have struggled to get their teenagers to appointments. We recommend taking time and helping your child to understand the wide range of benefits they'll enjoy as their mental health improves when they do seek help. Encourage your child to look at the opportunity for help from a big picture standpoint; you could weigh up the pros and cons together too. Reinforce in specific ways how life could be different with professional help. Sometimes, for stubborn teenagers, it's worth asking the question: 'What's it costing you not to go?'

In this chapter you'll learn what to expect during a visit to a general practitioner, how a mental health care plan will support you with costs, the importance of the psychologist–patient relationship and how a diagnosis can help.

## Anxious parents talking to anxious kids

Talking to a child about their anxiety symptoms is harder for some parents than others. It's especially hard if you have an anxiety disorder yourself. You may find that your own anxiety is triggered by what your child is going through. Perhaps you're reminded of your own experiences as a child or you become distressed now about a possible future. Their future. It's a perfectly natural by-product of the situation.

Anxious parents have told us that they've avoided talking about anxiety with their family, or even saying the word 'anxiety' around their children. One parent said she didn't want to give anxiety even a moment of 'air time', feeling as though the mere mention of it could bring it to life.

If you're feeling this way, take a moment to notice what you're thinking, and thank your mind for its concern (a defusion strategy) to create space between you and your thoughts. Take some deep breaths to calm your amygdala and then re-orient your attention back to what really matters. In this instance, what matters is opening up a conversation with your child if you haven't done so already.

## The start of an ongoing conversation

Start by sitting down for a chat to let them know you've noticed that they've been worried, that they don't want to do the activities they normally enjoy, that they're finding it hard to fall or stay asleep, that they are easily startled or more distracted or quiet than usual. Whatever it is you've noticed, there are many different ways you can open a conversation about anxiety. Here are a few you might choose to combine with the scripts we wrote for you in Chapter 3:

- Share some of your own worries from your childhood and ask your child if they've ever felt the same way.
- Mention what you've noticed and prompt your child to talk with you about what's going on for them: 'I noticed yesterday when Jamie asked if you wanted to go over to hang out, you didn't jump at the chance the way you normally would. I thought perhaps you didn't want to go at all. What were you thinking when that happened?'
- Ask about the worries they think about the most, or use an example of other children you know who have particular worries (maintaining their privacy at the same time): 'I know of another girl your age who worries a lot about being asked to answer a question in class. Do you ever feel like that too, about being asked a question by your teacher?'

Try to have a chat when they seem relaxed and content, you're not likely to be interrupted and you're both mentally present. It's reassuring for them to know you've noticed, to be reminded of how deeply you care about them, how you can help and who else can support them.

## Your anxious child's best friend – your local GP

We've all taken our children to the general practitioner once in a while for embarrassing check-ups. You'll know from experience that having a doctor your child feels comfortable with, trusts and is willing to open up to in the interests of their overall health and wellbeing is invaluable.

The same holds true if the time comes for a conversation about mental health. If your family doesn't yet have a GP that fits the bill, ask around other local parents or even check your local community Facebook page for recommendations. The Beyond Blue website is also a great resource for finding local health professionals. Take your time to find just the right person so that you both feel comfortable.

## Going alone or together?

Choosing to go to an initial appointment for a chat (with or without your partner) or together with your child will depend on a handful of factors, including:

- the age of your child
- your level of concern
- how long you've been curious or concerned
- if your child is asking for help
- the willingness of your child to seek help
- how you're coping with the situation.

When you go, start by explaining to the GP that you've come along to get some strategies to help with the symptoms you've noticed. The GP will take the lead from there.

You may find the GP reassures you that what you've observed is developmental and normal, and that you can expect the signs and symptoms to pass in due time. When children *are* anxious, it's often a huge relief for them to hear from their doctor that anxiety is common and well understood, that help is available and that they will get through this.

For teens aged fifteen and above, the GP will initially talk with the parent or carer and the teen so they have an opportunity to hear and validate concerns. Afterwards, the GP will talk with your teen on their own to build trust and offer privacy for a confidential conversation. If there are any concerns for your child's safety, the GP will let you know.

## What will the GP do to help?

A general practitioner will offer reassurance, a first assessment, helpful strategies and resources to support you and your anxious child from the first appointment. Anxiety symptoms can be connected to physical issues including, but not limited to, changes in the thyroid gland. The GP may investigate other possible underlying causes.

When needed, the GP will draft a mental health care plan and recommend access to psychological services under Medicare. Family therapy might be recommended for young children, whereas primary school children and adolescents could be referred to a psychologist for a type of 'talking' therapy. Your GP will help you to find a psychologist who is the right fit for your child. Ask all the questions you need answers to.

If your first appointment is a standard consultation, typically fifteen minutes, this initial meeting will help the GP to form a picture of what your child has been experiencing and how they're managing their symptoms. You may be asked to arrange another appointment to prepare the mental health care plan if deemed necessary. Alternatively, ask to book a longer appointment to begin with. The receptionist at the clinic will help you book the right appointment for your needs.

## Mental health care plans – better access to mental health professionals

The fees associated with professional help for anxiety will limit choices for some families whose budgets simply can't cover these additional and often unexpected costs.

To help Australians with the financial costs of seeking help for anxiety and other mental illnesses, the Better Access to Psychiatrists, Psychologists and General Practitioners through the Medicare Benefits Schedule, Better Access initiative was created by the Australian government. Better access means better outcomes. Mental health care plans are a central part of this initiative.

## So what does this mean for your child?

With a mental health care plan your child is entitled to attend up to ten appointments per year with an approved mental health professional, typically a psychologist. As their parent, you're entitled to a rebate from Medicare for some or all of the cost of each appointment, depending on the fees charged. The same applies if your child would benefit from group appointments and, in some cases, rebates are available for both individual and group appointments. The rebate also applies to the appointments you and your child attend with your general practitioner.

Eligible patients are entitled to a maximum of ten appointments, rebatable by Medicare, each calendar year but after the first six appointments you'll need to go back to your general practitioner with your child for a conversation about how the treatment is progressing. During this time the doctor will review the mental health care plan and information provided by the child's treating health professional and will prepare another referral for the remaining four appointments as needed.

Depending on the time of year the mental health care plan is prepared, how affordable professional services are for you, and the needs of your child, you can devise a plan with the child's psychologist, occupational therapist or other mental health professional to space out appointments in a way that fits with your child's treatment needs.

For instance, if your child's mental health care plan is devised in October, the ten appointments can be attended in the lead-up to the end of the calendar year. In the new year, a new mental health care plan can be prepared, entitling your child to another ten appointments over the following twelve months. This of course all depends on the professional assessment of both the treating mental health professional and the general practitioner.[1]

For some kids, a handful of appointments will make a profound difference to how they think and feel, others need more time. Your child's GP and mental health professional will incorporate you into your child's treatment plan and together you'll make the decisions that will be most helpful in teaching your child to manage their anxiety.

## Why finding a psychologist is like buying a pair of jeans

Whenever you go shopping for a pair of jeans, the first pair you try on isn't necessarily the last. It's a bonus if you get it right first time – the right colour denim, style, length and fit. Often you need to try on two pairs, sometimes more, to be confident that you've chosen the best pair to meet *your* needs and look great.

The same goes when choosing a psychologist. Unlike an electrician who will wire in a power point for you equally well whether you 'click' with them or not, or the dentist who is renowned for their excellent dental work and terrible bedside manner, when it comes to a psychologist, the relationship is paramount to the effectiveness of the treatment. A good 'fit' is everything.

## Mel's story

When Elise's daughter Mel was sixteen, she was diagnosed with anxiety and referred by her family doctor to see a local psychologist. A diagnosis brought incredible relief to Mel. She felt understood and optimistic for the first time in months.

A single parent, Elise joined Mel for the first psychology appointment. She helped share background information about Mel, how anxiety had been affecting her and how she'd been trying to help Mel to cope. Elise felt hopeful coming out of the appointment but Mel felt worse. She said the psychologist didn't understand her and that she didn't know what she was talking about. She was never going back.

Mel became despondent despite her optimism after being diagnosed. She was convinced that no one could help her. Not a psychologist, not her doctor, not her mum. Not surprisingly, this only fuelled more anxiety and distress.

Worries and anxiety can feel embarrassing. Feelings of guilt, shame or sadness that are hard for most kids to talk about will accompany anxiety for some kids. If your child doesn't form a good relationship with, and develop trust in, their psychologist, it may stand in the way of effective treatment.

If only Elise or Mel knew that they could go back to the doctor for a new referral to another reputable psychologist or one of their choice. If a GP hasn't had personal experience with a psychologist, they may be making a referral based on recommendations from their colleagues, their patients' experiences, location, convenience or availability.

Remember the jeans: the right pair for one child could be all wrong for another.

## Finding a great psychologist for your child

Founder of the Resilience Research Centre in Canada, family therapist and author Dr Michael Ungar has some great advice for parents when choosing a psychologist:

- The bond between the child and the psychologist is important. If there's a lack of trust or any reason your child isn't forming a connection with their psychologist, it's time to search for another one.
- A good psychologist recognises the child as a whole person, not merely as the product of their symptoms. They're able to separate the problem from the child and address it, while at the same time appreciating and drawing on the child's strengths.
- A good psychologist understands that they can best support a child by engaging and working with the child's parent, caregiver or guardian. They recognise that the special people already in the child's life are integral to the child's healing.
- Good psychologists don't claim to be the only source of support and help the child has available to them. They know in the long term that it's the child's social supports and family who make the biggest contribution to healing.
- A good psychologist understands the complexity of mental health challenges and recognises that attempting to attribute blame to the child or anyone else for the child's problem is at least unhelpful, and may potentially cause harm.
- Appreciating the culture of the child and of the child's caregivers is another way a good psychologist demonstrates their willingness to treat the whole person.[2]

## Explaining to your child how a psychologist will help

You're now in the process of getting your child's A-team together. They've most certainly got you, they've got their general practitioner and now they're about to add the jewel in the crown. While the time a psychologist spends with a child pales in comparison to the time you have with them, their contribution to your child's management of their anxiety is vital.

Teenagers are likely to understand the role of a psychologist to a certain extent, but might need their ideas extended. Psychologists help people who are experiencing serious challenges in their life, which could include change, stress, grief or financial problems. They also help people who are feeling anxious, depressed or are experiencing other mental illnesses.

It's helpful for a teen to know that a psychologist will assist them to understand more about their anxiety and the patterns that have developed around it, and help them develop thinking skills and lifestyle changes that positively impact anxiety symptoms and, moving forward, enable them to do all that's important to them, despite their anxiety.

Primary-school-aged children often benefit from hearing a psychologist's role described using an analogy. They understand that a doctor is the person to see if they're sick or injured, the dentist is the one to see for anything teeth-related and that the mechanic is the go-to place for car problems; so they can similarly understand the explanation that a psychologist is the professional who helps with thinking skills.

You're not alone if your child is less than keen to see a psychologist. Helping them understand the bigger picture of the benefits that come from getting the right support is a good way to nudge them in the direction towards help.

## How a diagnosis can help

It may take time for the exact nature of your child's anxiety to be clearly understood. A psychologist might meet with the parent for an initial appointment and will use early sessions with your child to ask questions so they can better understand how the anxiety is presenting, what's being done to manage it in both helpful and unhelpful ways, and how it's impacting on your child's life. While health professionals are often careful not to label kids, the right diagnosis lends itself to the right treatment approach.

## Your child is not their anxiety, no matter the diagnosis

Remember, whichever type of anxiety your child is diagnosed with, it doesn't change who they are and magnify their anxieties beyond what you've already been supporting them through. Picture your child as the most beautiful of blue skies – their anxieties are the clouds that float by. Sometimes there are a handful of fluffy white clouds, and sometimes the clouds are dark, stormy and plentiful.

An understanding of the nature of your child's anxiety is a wonderful step forward. Your child will always be the blue sky; their diagnosis will help everyone know how best to support them to watch the weather patterns come and go.

## 22

# Different approaches to managing and treating anxiety

Two effective approaches used by psychologists to treat anxious kids are cognitive behavioural therapy and acceptance and commitment therapy. The latter combines elements of cognitive behavioural therapy with mindfulness, acceptance, values, compassion and observation. Acceptance and commitment therapy underpins the understanding, tools, techniques and guides we've shared throughout this book.

## What therapy is (and isn't)

Thanks to Hollywood, most people picture 'therapy' as a psychologist sitting in an executive chair looking serious and taking notes, while the patient lies on a long couch answering questions about their childhood.

Let us reassure you, aside from the conversation, this is not what to expect for your child's treatment.

The conversation usually takes place in a comfortable and welcoming office or room where the psychologist and patient sit comfortably, sometimes with one or both parents there. Some psychologists will have a variety of objects and sensory toys for the child to hold or fiddle with during the appointment in the hope they find something that helps them feel more relaxed during the session. Teenagers often enjoy having something in their hands during a session too.

The relationship between the psychologist and patient is important. Time is taken to develop a level of trust and comfort so conversations flow freely and answers to questions come naturally. This will happen easily for some kids but take time for others.

## Cognitive behavioural therapy

The type of therapy most commonly used to treat children with anxiety disorders is cognitive behavioural therapy, or CBT. It's a talking therapy and has been widely researched for its effectiveness. In children, CBT is effective in almost 60 per cent of cases. The best evidence to date shows that when left untreated, only 16 per cent of children experience a natural decrease in their anxiety symptoms without any external support.[1]

CBT addresses the way kids think, feel and act. Central to CBT is the understanding that how we think and what we do affects how we feel, as represented below in the thoughts, feelings and behaviour triangle.

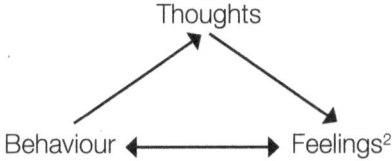

**Figure 2:** The thoughts, feelings, behaviour triangle

You'll know from experience how much your anxious child's thinking impacts how they feel and behave. An anxious child might have a thought about being onstage with the school band at the end-of-year concert (thought); a thought that almost instantaneously makes them feel upset and gives them a sick feeling in their stomach (feelings); prompting them to burst into tears and do all they can to avoid music lessons or rehearsals, or to want to quit music altogether (behaviours).

The goal of CBT is to support the child to develop skills, including:

- substituting more realistic or less frightening thoughts for ones that provoke anxiety
- relaxation
- gradual exposure to what makes them anxious
- finding evidence to dispute their thoughts.

The ultimate outcome is that the child changes their unhelpful or distorted thinking and dysfunctional behaviour, in turn changing how they feel.

## ERP or the stepladder approach

Exposure and response prevention (ERP) is one of the most important CBT techniques used with children. This is a type of 'face your fears' approach but it's not about throwing kids in the deep end. It's about breaking down an anxiety-provoking situation into small steps and supporting the anxious child to tolerate their anxiety with each exposure.

Also known as a stepladder approach, there might be anywhere between ten and twenty steps to move an anxious child towards a particular action.

For a child who becomes anxious around dogs, the first step might be to simply write the word 'dog' or look at a picture of a dog. Step by step, over time, the challenges become incrementally greater (and more anxiety-provoking) until the ultimate aim is achieved: patting or playing with a friendly dog.

Here's an example of a stepladder – also called the 'fear ladder' approach – for a child who is highly anxious around dogs:

| | |
|---|---|
| 1 | Write the word 'dog' |
| 2 | Play with a toy dog |
| 3 | Read a story about dogs |
| 4 | Look at photos of dogs |
| 5 | Look at videos of dogs, which are funny, silly or neutral |
| 6 | Watch a movie with dogs in it |
| 7 | Look at a dog through a window |
| 8 | Look at a group of dogs playing in a local park |
| 9 | Watch a dog playing in its front yard from across the road |
| 10 | Watch a (always friendly and trusted) dog on a leash from across the street |
| 11 | Stand 3 metres from a dog on a leash |
| 12 | Stand 2 metres from a dog on a leash |
| 13 | Stand 1 metre from a dog on a leash |
| 14 | Stand beside, but do not touch, a dog on a leash |
| 15 | Pat a puppy that someone else is holding |
| 16 | Hold a puppy |
| 17 | Pat a small dog on a leash |

| 18 | Pat a small dog off a leash |
|----|----------------------------|
| 19 | Pat a large dog on a leash |
| 20 | Pat a large dog off a leash[3] |

With every success along the way, the anxious child unlearns their instinctive avoidance behaviour. They'll also notice that they have the ability to tolerate the anxiety, which will inevitably start to fade the more they practise, giving them the courage to bravely take on the next step in their series of challenges. This is all done in a safe setting so the anxious child feels supported to do what feels hard. All the while they're moving in the direction of what's important to them.

For children diagnosed with obsessive-compulsive disorder (OCD), there can be up to fifty steps on a ladder for exposure and response prevention, because not only does the child need to tolerate the exposure (for instance, touching a doorhandle), they're also going to need to tolerate the added discomfort of avoiding their compulsion (perhaps washing their hands).

Steps to address these obsessions and compulsions could include a small and brief exposure to 'germs' followed by a small reduction in handwashing time and the amount of soap used, or number of repetitions of handwashing.

## What about medication?

Medication for children for any illness – physical or mental – is a question to consider carefully as a parent. Anxiety medication is prescribed by a general practitioner or a psychiatrist. The decision to medicate a child or teen depends on a number of factors. While some research shows medication is an effective way of treating anxiety,[4] questions remain unanswered. A safe age to begin treatment is not clear; nor is a depth of understanding and management of medication side effects, the most effective duration of treatment, dependency issues and the impact of stopping anti-anxiety mediation on children.[5]

When asked on SBS *Insights*' 'Beating Anxiety' episode for his thoughts on medication, Director of Coaching and Positive Psychology at Macquarie University John Franklin suggested we consider how anxiety affects the whole person. Though his comments centred on medication for adults, his thoughts were insightful for parents of anxious children. He reiterated that anxiety wasn't just a psychological and cognitive process, that it was a process that also brought about physical changes. He saw two circumstances under which medication could be useful:

> The first is that many times people's anxiety is in part the result of them having a very overactive, very reactive nervous system . . . it can sometimes be useful to dampen that whole thing down. Medication can be useful there.

He noted a second situation that can be more common: people are so agitated that they can't think properly. 'They can't think clearly, they can't make sense of a situation and take useful and corrective action. In that situation reducing the level of agitation to the point where people can rethink their life, make effective decisions and take appropriate actions is very helpful.'

He added that generally speaking one should try to take medication at minimal effective doses for as short a time as possible. This advice applies to all ages of patients taking anxiety medication.

## When the solution becomes the problem

Anxiety feels awful. It follows then that anxious kids work hard to avoid feeling anxious any way they can. Now we've introduced you to the thoughts, feelings, behaviour triangle, it's easy to see how the solution can become the problem.

Here's an example:

Thoughts      I can't perform in the concert, I'll freeze onstage
              and embarrass myself.

Feelings      Sick to the stomach, sweaty, dizzy and emotional

Behaviours    Not going to music lessons, teary

Thoughts      I'm hopeless, if I can't even get to my music lessons
              there's no way I'll be able to perform at the concert.
              I might as well just give up now.

Feelings      Sad, hopeless, overwhelmed

Behaviour     Cancels lessons altogether

You can see from this example how a negative cycle develops, how behaviours in turn impact on thinking, and how what feels like the solution becomes a part of the problem.

Here's another example:

Thoughts      I can't go away on the surf camp – how will I cope for
              four nights so far away without my parents around
              me? I know something will happen to them.

Feelings      Disappointed, hopeless, weird, lonely, worried

Behaviour     Cancels surf camp

Thoughts      They won't miss me if I don't go to camp.
              Why would they?

              They think I'm a baby because I don't want to go on camp.

              The other kids will probably be glad I'm not going.

Feelings      Disgusted, regretful, sad, defeated

Behaviour     More avoidance

When the solution becomes the problem, life becomes more difficult, not less. Acceptance and commitment therapy is a psychological treatment that helps anxious people overcome these vicious cycles.

## Acceptance and commitment therapy (ACT)

Professor Steve Hayes from the University of Nevada pioneered acceptance and commitment therapy, which is pronounced ACT (the word, not the letters A-C-T). He notes that CBT is also evidence-based. 'If you're doing that with exposure (ERP) with a competent person and it's working for you, please do that,' he says. As for ACT, he points out that it's 'part of the family of CBTs. Traditional CBT had this idea that you had to change the form of your thinking in order to change the form of your feeling so that you could behave differently. What ACT asks you to do is change your relationship to your thinking, change your relationship to your feeling and get about the business of living life now.'

The aim of ACT is different to that of CBT. CBT aims to teach children to:

1. Recognise their anxious thoughts. For example: 'My freckle is a skin cancer.'
2. Find evidence to challenge the accuracy of their thoughts. For example: 'I've had that freckle for years, it's always the same'; 'I'm fit and well'; 'It's not sore'; 'It would look different if there was really a problem'; 'My doctor told me it's okay.'
3. Replace their anxious thoughts with more realistic, hopeful and encouraging ones. For example: 'It's nothing to worry about, I'm healthy, it's just another freckle.'

The aim of ACT is to change the relationship with thoughts and feelings so they're no longer viewed as symptoms but as uncomfortable events that come and go. The underlying philosophy is developing acceptance for unwanted thoughts, worries, bodily sensations and feelings and then taking action to move in the direction of what's truly valued.[6]

Dr Russ Harris, author of the international bestseller *The Happiness Trap*, talks about acceptance of thoughts and feelings and taking values-guided action. He says that despite our difficult and painful thoughts and feelings, our arms and legs continue to move, meaning that we are still capable of continuing on with our lives. We don't have to wait until our anxiety has passed, or we feel great, to do what matters. The aim of ACT is not to rid ourselves of our anxiety, but to live a rich, full, colourful and meaningful life with it. The reality is that anxiety stays with us but it doesn't have to stop us doing what's important and what brings us closer to our cherished goals. We can turn the dial on anxiety to low and take it along for the ride.

## The principles of ACT

There are six core ACT principles that foster psychological flexibility – the ability to mindfully bring your attention to the present moment and to take values-guided action. ACT principles are peppered throughout this book to skill you up in order to support your anxious child.

The core principles of ACT are:

1. acceptance
2. defusion
3. being present
4. self as context (observing thoughts and feelings)
5. values
6. committed action.

ACT itself is a flexible psychological intervention, as skill development can begin with any of the six core principles. There are great resources available to further support your learning. Visit www.actmindfully.com.au to explore Dr Harris's resources and workshops.

## The struggle is real

There's a great deal of struggle with anxiety. The way it feels prompts people to want to get rid of any difficult thoughts and feelings. However, the more they struggle with avoiding a thought or a feeling, the more grief it brings. The same holds true for anxious kids.

An ACT approach helps children learn to notice their thoughts but to relate to them in a new way: by noticing them, but not engaging with them. All thoughts and feelings come and go; what matters is taking action to keep moving in the direction of important values. Going to the movies with friends, playing sport, playing an instrument in the school band, going on camp, having a sleepover at a friend's house, going to school, sitting a test and going to sports training are all examples of taking action in the direction of what's important, despite any anxiety that shows up.

The two main goals of ACT are:

1. fostering acceptance of unwanted thoughts and feelings whose occurrence or disappearance cannot be controlled
2. commitment and action towards living a life they value.[7]

ACT helps children develop the skills to accept their thoughts and feelings, to accept themselves and others with compassion, to know what matters to them (what they value) and to commit to actions that move them in those directions.[8]

Psychologists all over the world are training in ACT to broaden their treatment options for clients. You don't have to be a psychologist to undertake the training. You too can undertake training in ACT, developing your own understanding of the model to support your child to manage their anxiety in parallel with the other health professionals on your child's team.

# 23

# How schools can help

School can be a challenging place for a student who's prone to experiencing anxiety. A familiar teacher's absence, a large group-learning activity, taking part in competitive sport or auditioning for the school play are the sorts of everyday activities that can make an anxious child's pulse race, their thoughts wander and their stomach churn. School is a hotbed of anxious moments for many students.

A child's anxiety, if unmanaged, almost always interferes with learning. It's difficult for a student to concentrate if they're worried or anxious about a future event. Lack of concentration can also be compounded by fear – fear of failure, fear of rejection, fear of being laughed at – which causes a student to take safe learning options or, worse, to avoid participating in activities that make them feel anxious. Alternatively, fear can drive a student to over-plan, over-rehearse or over-train to ensure success, which is exhausting. An anxious student may achieve socially, academically or in other areas of school life, but success can come at the cost of happiness, wellbeing and mental health, either now or in the future. Anxiety, left unchecked, generally catches up with students eventually.

## Actions schools can take

In our experience, teachers are worried about the current anxiety epidemic that's impacting students. Many teachers are fully aware that something, namely anxiety, is impacting student learning and behaviour, but they are unsure of its nature or how they can help. This is not a criticism, as a teacher's inability to fully understand the nature of anxiety is a reflection of the wider community's confusion when it comes to the issue. Fortunately, there is much teachers can do both to minimise anxiety in the first place and, importantly, to assist kids to regulate and manage anxiousness when it occurs.

## Understand and normalise anxiety

Anxiety is an emotional term. Most people grimace at the very mention of the word. In reality, anxiety is not a condition to fear, or demonise. It's part of a gamut of emotions that everyone experiences; however, some children experience it at far greater levels than others. As we've discussed, there is more in the current environment – such as increased digital technology, sedentary lifestyles and poor sleep patterns – to turn anxiety on in kids' brains than at any other time in recent history.

Over the last decade many high-profile sportspeople in Australia have publicly acknowledged the impact that anxiety has had on their mental health and performance. Anxiety's impact has been so challenging that sportspeople such as cricketer Moises Henriques, AFL footballer Lance Franklin and netballer Sharni Layton have had to take time away from their sports to restore their mental health. The public admissions of their anxiety experiences and those of other high-profile sports stars has helped to normalise anxiety, reinforcing the fact that no one is immune and, importantly, that there should be no shame attached.

A teacher can help normalise anxiety by speaking about it in everyday terms in the classroom. By talking about anxiety matter-of-factly a teacher can send the message to their students that anxiousness doesn't need to be hidden. Talking about it reinforces the message that anxiety is experienced by many people and can be successfully managed.

The normalisation process is enhanced when a teacher builds their self-awareness about their own anxiety. Knowing the activities that make them anxious as a teacher helps build empathy and understanding when a student becomes anxious or worried about an activity that many other students would embrace or approach with nonchalance. Reflecting on their own coping and management skills also puts a teacher in a good position to help an anxious child.

It's easy for teachers to miss anxiety if student behaviour is their focus. Anxiousness can typically result in avoidance or perfectionism, which are behaviours that most teachers are familiar with. Anxiety can sometimes show as anger and frustration, which are completely different emotions. When a teacher is on the lookout for anxiety it's easier to see the emotion behind behaviour and to recognise it even when it's hiding behind anger's noisy, in-your-face mask.

## Adapt a common approach to managing anxiety

Like taking a pill that eases the symptoms without treating the condition behind it, avoidance is a key strategy that kids use to ease their anxiety. The symptoms may fade or disappear, but the condition remains and will show next time they meet a similar situation.

We encourage teachers to help students accept their anxiety as being a common reaction to a potentially challenging situation. However, rather than practising avoidance to ease discomfort, a student should gradually be exposed to the situation or event that makes them anxious. This may take time, sensitivity and patience, which can be in short supply in busy classrooms. A teacher's willingness to work one-on-one with an anxious student, gradually exposing them to an anxiety-inducing situation, will help the student in the long run.

## Validate rather than reassure

Anxious students frequently look to their teachers to provide reassurance when they feel anxious. The need for reassurance shows in many ways, including kids continually seeking a teacher's opinion, wanting the teacher to make decisions for them, and continually asking for praise. It's acceptable to offer some reassurance when a student is anxious; however, too much reassurance can lead to student dependency on teachers and other adults to manage or prevent feelings of anxiety.

Anxious children may seek reassurance, but validation of their anxiousness is preferable to reassurance. We suggest that teachers use 'Ahhhh' statements to validate how an anxious student is feeling, which shows them they're listening and trying to understand. Here are some examples:

'Ahhhh, you're feeling anxious about going to school camp . . .'

'Ahhhh, you're having one of those "I might mess it up" thoughts . . .'

'Ahhhh, you're feeling disappointed that didn't work out for you . . .'

## Help students stepladder their way out of anxiousness

Stepladdering is a technique with wide application at school. Rather than allowing students to avoid challenging situations we encourage teachers to look for ways to incrementally challenge students to achieve what really matters to them at school.

### Sophie's story

Nine-year-old Sophie feared group work in the classroom. When children were placed into groups of four for co-operative activities, Sophie always refused to join in. Unsure how she should respond, Sophie's teacher, Mrs Turner, allowed Sophie to work on her own rather than join others. After four different group work sessions in which Sophie worked alone, Mrs Turner decided that avoidance wasn't helping. A change of tack was needed. Mrs Turner used step-laddering, also known as exposure and response prevention (ERP), to gradually familiarise Sophie with group work. Mrs Turner and Sophie set the long-term goal of Sophie being able to work comfortably with any group of students in the class. But first she had to take small steps up the step-ladder to group work success.

Initially, Sophie worked with her friend Eli during small group activities. She worked well with Eli and felt comfortable in her company. When Mrs Turner was satisfied that Sophie could work well with Eli, she then moved Sophie up a step on the ladder and gave Sophie a different partner to work with during group sessions. Sophie was soon comfortable with this arrangement, so Mrs Turner asked Sophie to work in a group of four, consisting of Eli and two other students she'd worked with before. Sophie was also given the simple job of being a timekeeper, responsible for keeping the group on task. This was one more step up the ladder to success-ful group work for Sophie. Mrs Turner saw that Sophie was comfortable with this arrangement, so during the next group work session she wasn't given a specific role but was asked to join in all activities. As Sophie felt comfortable working with this group, she was able to contribute and follow instruc-tions provided by the group leader. This arrangement stood for several sessions. Sophie was one step away from what they had predetermined was to be their goal. The final step was for Sophie to work with at least three other students she hadn't worked with before. Sophie achieved this last task easily. Within a few months Sophie had gone from shyness and avoidance to happily working with others using this exposure and response prevention technique.

## Teach students how anxiety works

In Chapter 3 we explained how important it is for kids to understand how anxiety impacts their brains and their bodies. This self-knowledge demystifies anxiety and helps kids recognise and manage their anxious states. For instance, a child who fully understands the calming impact that mindfulness can have on the amygdala is more likely to use this potent tool than one who has no understanding of the relationship between the two. We also provided some scripts that parents can use to explain how the anxious brain works and the impact of anxiety on a child's physiology.

Teachers, with greater expertise and resources at hand, can support these scripts with more in-depth psychoeducation sessions in the classroom. Hearing this, many teachers may think, 'Not something else that teachers have to teach kids. The curriculum is crowded already and I don't have the expertise.' We don't wish to add to teachers' workload; however, by teaching kids how an anxious brain works, they provide students with a valuable reference point to help them self-manage their anxiety. The use of a common language is also an invaluable asset in a child's anxiety management. Whether such information is delivered as part of a broader science curriculum, or comes under the heading of social and emotional learning, teaching kids how their brains and bodies react to stress is the type of education that will help them be successful beyond the school gate and in any work environment imaginable.

## Make classrooms psychologically safe

Every teacher knows that a safe classroom is necessary for optimum learning, but this goes beyond physical safety. Students also need to feel psychologically safe if they are to prosper at school.

### Ready, set, test

Mr X suddenly announced to his Year Nine class that everyone would sit an unexpected test in two days' time. This announcement received mixed student reactions. A small number who thrived on test situations gave internal high fives and thought, 'Bring it on!' The majority were annoyed that the test came out of the blue, but realising such was school life thought, 'I've got two days to prepare. Hopefully that will be enough.' A small number went into panic mode. Three students sat staring into space, while one student angrily remonstrated with the teacher about a lack of preparation time. This group thought, 'Oh no. I can't do this.' This latter group's response is typical of many anxious students, whose brains will do anything to help them feel safe. The sudden announcement of a test took them by surprise, affecting their psychological need for control. When they didn't feel in control they felt unsafe and their amygdala took over from their prefrontal cortex. So flight, fight or freeze became their first response.

Mr X had no intention of making his students feel unsafe – he wanted to challenge them academically. However, his announcement of a test without prior warning and with little preparation time violated the need for all his students to feel psychologically safe. The anxious brain can't differentiate between a real physical threat or a psychological threat. Physiologically they are the same, so those students responded to the impending test in the same way as they would to a threat of being physically hurt.

There are common features of psychologically safe classrooms that anxious students need, which we will discuss below.

## Authoritative leadership

Classrooms suit anxiety-prone students when they are led by teachers who use an authoritative leadership style. Authoritative leaders, first identified by science journalist Daniel Goleman in his theory of emotional intelligence, are able to relate individually to others while maintaining a sense of order or authority. They differ from authoritarian leaders in that they are less concerned with obedience and rigid sticking to rules and more concerned with individual differences and, at the same time, they are able to maintain an orderly environment. A teacher's ability to maintain an orderly classroom environment is paramount if an anxious child is to feel safe at school.

## Structure, regularity and routine

Students who are prone to anxiety thrive on structure, regularity and routine. The first thought for many anxious children when they wake is: 'What will my day look like?' They will invariably run the day through their predictability lens; if there are no surprises ahead, then they will feel comfortable. If there is uncertainty or doubt, such as indecision about who is picking them up after school, they'll feel tense or anxious. If they have an excursion that they haven't been well prepared for the change of routine will invariably leave them feeling nervous and tense. Anxious kids, like groups, function best when they can successfully predict and prepare for what's ahead. They love classrooms that are well-organised, well-led and structured in a way that allows them to predict the types of activities and lessons that will occur at any given time.

## Social storytelling

As the understanding and awareness of autism grows, many teachers are finding that they have numerous students diagnosed with autism in their class. They will most likely be well aware that any change in daily structure or routine will be the cause of a great deal of anxiety for students on the autism spectrum. As we outlined earlier, social storytelling, or talking kids through new situations, is a wonderful way to prepare a child with autism for a potentially stressful event. This strategy can also be used to prepare all students for new or unusual scenarios. For instance, before going on an excursion a teacher can talk students through the possible day, including as much detail as is practical, such as visual information to help students access the visual parts of their brain, which will help them mentally map out the day ahead.

## Individual student self-management plans

Students who have successfully returned to school following school refusal generally have done so as a result of a joint management plan involving teachers, parents and carers and the student, often with professional input. These plans usually incrementally expose a student to more elements of school, such as classwork done at home, being driven to school without getting out of the car, and meeting friends after school in the school grounds as they start to feel comfortable. This strategy can be extended to other situations in which students display anxiety. A student who refuses to go onstage in the school play can work as a stagehand; then their contribution may be extended to being part of a crowd scene. Similarly, an individual anxiety management plan can be designed to assist a student who is anxious about going to school camp by starting with attending the camp for half a day, then extending to a full day and so on. Alternatively, a parent could stay overnight on the camp but keep a distance to allow their anxious child to develop independence with the knowledge that comfort is close by if needed. It's important to involve a student in the formulation of an individual management plan as they need to feel that they are in control of their plan. As soon as they feel that exposure will escalate against their will or beyond their capacity to cope, the best-laid plan is invariably doomed to failure.

## Incorporate anxiety management tools into school and classroom life

Teachers, like parents, can give kids in their care the tools they need to self-regulate their anxiety so they aren't reliant on others to ease their anxiousness. In Part 4 we introduced in detail five key self-regulation tools that parents can use. These can also be incorporated in classroom and school life. Here's how.

### Checking in

'How do you feel about the school formal?' Now that's a question that will elicit all sorts of responses, from 'nervous', 'happy', 'jittery' or 'excited' to 'fantastic', 'awesome' or 'toey'. They're all legitimate responses that indicate different levels of emotional awareness. 'I don't know' is the non-preferred response as this indicates a lack of emotional awareness. If students are to adequately regulate their anxiousness, they need to build their awareness of their emotional states. Some students will do this quite naturally, while others will genuinely struggle to identify the many and varied feelings that may be impacting them at any given time. For these reasons we recommend that all students are taught a method to identify their emotions. Our preferred method – checking in – is outlined in Chapter 9 and is easy for teachers to integrate into classroom life. It's also a useful tool that helps teachers to support their students to shift into moods helpful for successfully completing different learning tasks. For example, a student will benefit from moving into a reflective mood to complete an analytic writing task. Checking in with emotions is the first step in this task for a student.

## Exercise

Exercise is one of the best ways to release the tension and stress caused by anxiety. Exercise that successfully releases tension involves the large limbs – the arms and legs. Simple playground activities involving running, chasing and climbing are generally sufficient to release nervous tension and encourage feel-good endorphins to flow. However, not every child will run around during recess, many preferring to sit and play quiet games. Anecdotal evidence suggests that secondary school students move around a great deal less than primary school students, so teachers may have to be proactive to get students moving.

There are many ways schools can get students moving, ranging from a commitment from all teachers to incorporate some type of movement into regular lessons; daily exercise or movement activities that involve the whole school or year levels, such as starting the day with games, and movement to music or dance; or encouraging students to walk or ride bikes to school.

## Mindfulness and breathing

Schools require students to constantly look ahead to the next day, the next week and the next term. Anxiety is felt in the present but is often future driven. Tomorrow's homework, next week's swimming lessons and next term's camp can all drive anxiety to the extent that some students spend all their time worrying, ruminating and fretting about activities that haven't even happened yet.

The daily practice of mindfulness is a wonderful way to bring students' attention back to the present. We recommend that teachers not only use mindfulness with students when they become stressed, but also incorporate it into everyday school and classroom life. Mindfulness can be combined with movement, but it almost always combines with deep breathing. Starting a learning session with a three- to five-minute mindfulness activity can be a wonderful way to set the mood for a session of learning, as well as teaching a helpful calming tool to kids. Also, the incorporation of simple breathing activities into class sessions demonstrates to students simple relaxation techniques they can call on at any time.

### Defusion

Here's the most potent question a teacher can ask a student who's worrying about a future event: 'Are these worries or thoughts helpful?' Invariably the answer will be no, leading to the next question: 'What can you do that's helpful?' It's crucial that teachers encourage kids to step back and consider their thinking in an analytical way. This enables students to look *at* their thoughts instead of *from* them. Parents can do this within the family context, but teachers have a more rounded educational context in which they can encourage students to notice and reflect on their thoughts. The distancing technique outlined in Chapter 13, in which kids catch their negative thought patterns, such as 'I'll do poorly in that test', before adding a phrase like 'I notice I had a thought that I'll do poorly in that test', is an example of a defusion technique that can be taught to students of most ages. After a student has identified their thinking as unhelpful, the next step is encouraging them to take action, to do something that leads them in a valued direction.

## Traffic light wellbeing plan

A simple, effective tool teachers can use to raise student's awareness of their wellbeing is the traffic light wellbeing plan. Used in hospital settings, nutrition, aged-care and mental health, the traffic light system is an almost universally understood approach for making evaluations. With a personal traffic light wellbeing plan, students can enter details into each section to describe how they feel and what they do when they're feeling good, when they're beginning to struggle and when they are indeed struggling and need help.

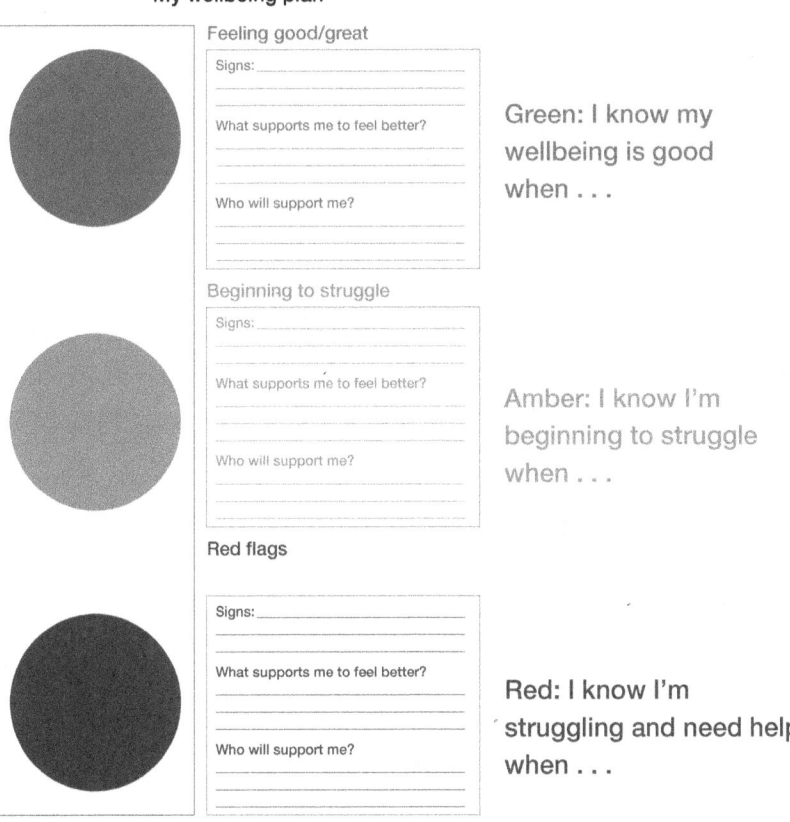

**My wellbeing plan**

Feeling good/great

Signs: _____

What supports me to feel better?

Who will support me?

Green: I know my wellbeing is good when . . .

Beginning to struggle

Signs: _____

What supports me to feel better?

Who will support me?

Amber: I know I'm beginning to struggle when . . .

Red flags

Signs: _____

What supports me to feel better?

Who will support me?

Red: I know I'm struggling and need help when . . .

**Figure 3:** Traffic light wellbeing plan

Using the traffic light wellbeing plan:

1. Open a conversation with students about feelings. All feelings are natural, they come and they go; some feel good and some don't. There are no wrong feelings, and it's natural to experience a range of feelings every day. Introduce students to the thoughts, feelings, behaviour triangle from Chapter 22 so they can begin to develop an understanding of how each affects another. You could share the example included in that chapter to illustrate the point. You could extend this activity to include a class (or pairs or small group) brainstorm of feelings and then list or collate them on the board.

2. Ask students to contribute to a group discussion about their thoughts, feelings and behaviour when they're feeling good. Prompt students to think about their sleep, their mood, how much they exercise, how sociable they feel, what they do for fun, how they feel during class and while completing homework, who they like to spend time with, their participation in after-school activities, how they feel, the content of their thoughts and self-talk, choices related to their health and how much time they spend on screens. Note all of these on a whiteboard under the heading 'Feeling good', written in green if possible. Anxious students may find a group discussion challenging; tweak this activity as needed to meet the needs of your students.

3. Distribute a wellbeing plan to each student and ask them to complete the green 'Feeling good' section using some of the class examples they relate to and others that are unique to their experiences. Allow time for items to be included by each student. Students can then include details of what supports them to continue to feel good, helping them stay in the green zone of their wellbeing plan.

4. Repeat step 2 for the next (amber) section 'Beginning to struggle', compiling class answers on the whiteboard under that same heading, preferably written in orange.

5. Ask students to complete the amber section of their personal plan. This section has a space for them to also include the action(s) they can take to help move them from the amber zone towards the green zone. They can note the names of people they can turn to for support if they're beginning to struggle. This list could include parents, other family members, a particular teacher or even their family doctor. Encourage them to be specific.

6. The 'Red flags' zone of the wellbeing plan can be completed in the same manner as the amber zone. This is an opportunity to chat with the class about symptoms of declining wellbeing, including social withdrawal, low mood most of the time, heightened anxiety, difficulty falling or staying asleep, making poor food choices or spending a lot of time in front of a screen. They might feel irritable, sad, stressed or angry a lot of the time; they might feel guilty, miserable, frustrated, unhappy or disappointed most of the time. They might have an upset stomach, feel shaky or overwhelmed; they might worry about school, friendships, family or their future; they may avoid activities they usually enjoy or find it difficult to concentrate. Use age-appropriate examples during each step to ensure you're facilitating discussions at the right level for the students in your class.

7. Create a regular opportunity for students to reflect on their plan and to choose which colour best represents their level of wellbeing at that time. Encourage students to put their plan into action by undertaking the actions they listed that will support them to move towards the green zone when needed.

## Teachers practise what they preach

In recent years there have been numerous reports highlighting the stressful nature of teaching. A 2017 report into the impact of stress on Australian teachers showed that one in eighty-three teachers is on long-term stress or mental health leave.[1] This is an increase of 5 per cent in one year. Another report revealed that 20 per cent of teachers considered changing careers in the first five years of teaching due to high levels of stress and burnout. The story is the same in other parts of the world, with 93 per cent of elementary teachers in the US state of Missouri reporting high levels of stress.[2] There's no doubt that school is a stressful workplace. Teachers are notorious for putting their own welfare behind that of their students, many working long hours and tackling a variety of tasks that they feel ill-equipped or simply too stretched to manage.

If the anxiety epidemic is to be tackled comprehensively in schools, it's imperative that teachers attend to their own mental health and wellbeing. It's difficult for a teacher who is constantly stressed to give students the assistance they need. While teacher stress needs to be tackled in a holistic way, including managing workloads, improving student behaviour and providing sufficient time to implement new skills, there is much teachers can do to manage their own stress.

The five anxiety management tools outlined in Part 4 – checking in, deep breathing, mindfulness, exercise and defusion – provide a wonderful platform for the management of teacher anxiety. We urge teachers to add these tools to their personal wellbeing repertoires so their use becomes routine, enabling them to draw on these strategies in response to their own anxiety. We know from our research and experience the positive impact these tools can have on a person's effectiveness and happiness, and we feel confident that they will help teachers to be more empathetic and better able to respond to the varied needs of students. Additionally, it's hard to teach a personal skill to kids when you don't use it yourself. A teacher who understands how mindfulness works is more likely to introduce it into their class. A teacher who has experienced how quickly deep breathing switches on their relaxation response also knows how it can quickly change the mood in a class. A teacher who has experienced the release of tension that exercise brings is more likely to look for opportunities to get kids moving at school. When teachers practise what they teach, their passion and intent shows through, making it easier for students to latch on to these important anxiety management techniques.

# Epilogue

Anxiety is personal. When someone close to you experiences anxiety you feel an array of unpleasant and often difficult emotions, including worry, confusion, apprehension and anguish. We hope that by reading this book you now experience a sense of relief, assurance and comfort. Relief that the anxiety experienced by the child or children in your life is common and well understood. Assurance that a greater understanding of anxiety, a practical set of tools and a healthy lifestyle will enable an anxious child to live a full and happy life. And most of all, comfort in the fact that you are not alone on your journey assisting kids to move from anxiety into resilience. Hopefully, like us, you feel a sense of excitement to be part of a movement of people who are helping to change community attitudes, where questions and conversations about anxiety are seen as normal, and anxiety is no longer viewed as an affliction or a topic to be avoided or only talked about behind closed doors. We also hope you are excited to be at the vanguard of a significant change to the way that we manage anxiety in children and young people.

## Accept and commit

Anxiety may be a constant companion for many kids, but it's certainly not their best friend. Often, it's a demon with which they are locked in a long-running, laborious battle where simple activities such as attending school camp become something they dread. Alternatively, they ignore anxiety altogether and avoid events or situations that bring discomfort. 'No way. I'm not getting involved,' becomes their default as they set limits on their potential and their happiness.

We advocate that kids accept their anxiety rather than fight it or ignore it and hope it goes away. Usually anxiety doesn't dissipate. If left unmanaged, the symptoms may disappear for a time but will typically recur in later childhood or in adulthood. We want kids to face up to their fears and commit to doing whatever is important to them, despite their feelings of anxiety. The child who would love to perform onstage, but avoids auditioning for a school play owing to their anxiety is missing so much. It's better that they accept that performing in the play brings about anxiety but go ahead and participate anyway, using some of the tools outlined in this book to help them manage their emotional state. It helps immensely if they have a supportive parent, teacher or coach who recognises the turmoil their anxiety causes, but who encourages them every step of the way to take part and engage in activities and manage their anxiety as it ebbs and flows. While this accept and commit approach may not initially bring a child comfort, their anxiety will eventually decrease as they become more adept at moving it to the background while engaging in activities that bring with them meaning, purpose and joy.

## Putting the learning into practice

It can be difficult knowing where to start when you want to help a child. We suggest you resist the urge to make wholesale changes to the way you currently assist kids to manage their anxiousness.

Just as many New Year's resolutions hastily made in January are often discarded in February, revolutionary-type behavioural change rarely lasts. A graded approach – in which small, incremental changes and improvements are made – is more effective and long-lasting.

## Talk about it

Discuss what you have learned in this book with a partner, colleague or friend. This will help you to synthesise the ideas and strategies you've discovered that are relevant to your situation. Verbalisation will assist you to clarify and order your thoughts, bringing to the surface those ideas that are most important to you. By discussing the contents of this book you may even enlist a trusted ally to support you to make changes within your family, classroom or group to better support the anxious child in your life.

## Keep change manageable

Break down the skills and tools you want to implement into manageable chunks. Start by responding thoughtfully rather than reacting automatically when a child catastrophises or overreacts to a situation or event. Don't worry if at first you don't know what to say to a child who thinks the world is about to end. Focus on staying calm via your breathing and notice how the anxiety dance might be playing out in that moment. Focusing on your own actions is a wonderful place to start when achieving behavioural change in others.

## Bring kids along with you

In age-appropriate ways, create open dialogue with the kids in your life about anxiety. Help them understand the physiological basis of anxiety so they can become better self-managers of their own emotions. Discuss the events and situations that usually trigger anxiety so they can consciously (rather than unconsciously) prepare themselves to react, or in some cases, overreact. Share with kids your own fears, worries and anxieties and discuss the coping mechanisms that you've found work for you. Healthy families and groups function well on the premise that there is nothing so bad that happens that people can't talk about it. Being open doesn't encourage a child's anxiety. It helps create a culture of acceptance, normalisation and empathy.

## Strike when the iron is cold

Don't wait until the child is in the middle of a panic attack to introduce a tool such as deep breathing to calm them down. Instead, practise deep breathing in fun ways when they are calm and have their emotions under control. The same principle applies with other tools outlined in this book, especially mindfulness and defusion which are more challenging to implement under stress. Tools that rescue kids when they are anxious need to be practised repeatedly in low-stress situations so they can be easily accessed when needed.

## Stay with us

This book is the start of a journey to better manage the anxiety of the kids in your life. Like you, we want kids to find success and happiness, with all that they love taking centre stage in their lives, and their anxiety relegated to the wings. We invite you to continue the journey you've begun with this book. Our exploration of helping kids turn anxiety into resilience continues and we'd love to share our discoveries with you. We'd also like to hear about your challenges and, importantly, your successes using the approach, tools and lifestyle factors that we've advocated in this book. The following page contains our details where you can join with us as we continue to explore practical ways to help anxious kids live life in full colour.

# Appendix

## Stay connected with Michael and Jodi

### *Reach Michael online*

Website: www.parentingideas.com.au

Facebook: Parenting Ideas

Twitter: @michaelgrose

Blog: www.parentingideas.com.au/blog

Schools: www.parentingideas.com.au/schools

### Reach Jodi online

Website: www.drjodirichardson.com.au

Facebook: Dr Jodi Richardson – Happier on Purpose

Instagram: @drjodirichardson

Twitter: @DrJodiR

Blog: drjodirichardson.com.au/blog

# Notes

## Chapter 1

1. Gregory, A. M., Caspi, A., Moffitt, T. E., Koenen, K., Eley, T. C. & Poulton, R., 'Juvenile mental health histories of adults with anxiety disorders', *American Journal of Psychiatry*, 164(2), 2007, pp. 301–8.

2. Chris McCurry shared this viewpoint in 2017 during an interview for our Parenting Anxious Kids online course (www.parentingideas.com.au/product/parenting-anxious-kids-online-course).

3. Polanczyk, G. V., Salum, G. A., Sugaya, L. S., Caye, A. & Rohde, L. A., 'Annual research review: A meta-analysis of the worldwide prevalence of mental disorders in children and adolescents', *Journal of Child Psychology and Psychiatry*, 56(3), 2015, pp. 345–65.

4. Young Minds Matter Mental Health Survey, 2015.

5. Australian Institute of Health and Welfare, 'Australia's Health 2018: In brief', 2018.

6. Twenge, J. M., Gentile, B., DeWall, C.N., Ma, D., Lacefield, K., Schurtz, D., 'Birth cohort increases in psychopathology among young Americans, 1938–2007', *Clinical Psychology Review*, 30, 2010.

7. Twenge, J. M., 'The age of anxiety? The birth cohort change in anxiety and neuroticism, 1952–1993', *Journal of Personality and Social Psychology*, 79(6), 2000, pp. 1007–21.

8. Xin, Z., Zhang, L. & Liu, D., 'Birth cohort changes of Chinese adolescents' anxiety: A cross-temporal meta-analysis, 1992–2005', *Personality and Individual Differences*, 48(2), 2010, pp. 208–12; National Society for the Prevention of Cruelty to Children, 'Anxiety a rising concern in young people contacting Childline', 2016.

9. Hiscock, H., Neely, R. J., Lei, S. & Freed, G., 'Paediatric mental and physical health presentations to emergency departments, Victoria, 2008–15', *Medical Journal of Australia*, 208(8), 2018, pp. 343–8.

10. Ialongo, N., Edelsohn, G., Werthamer-Larsson, L., Crockett, L. & Kellam, S., 'The significance of self-reported anxious symptoms in first-grade children', *Journal of Abnormal Child Psychology*, 22(4), 1994, pp. 441–55.

11. Bhatia, M. S. & Goyal, A., 'Anxiety disorders in children and adolescents: Need for early detection', *Journal of Postgraduate Medicine*, 64(2), 2018, pp. 75–6.

12. Kessler R. C., Berglund, P., Demler, O., Jin, R., Merikangas, K. R. & Walters, E. E., 'Lifetime prevalence and age-of-onset distributions of DSM-IV disorders in the National Comorbidity Survey Replication', *Archives of General Psychiatry*, 62(6), 2005, p. 593.

13. Leutwyler, B., 'Metacognitive learning strategies: Differential development patterns in high school', *Metacognition and Learning*, 4(2), 2009, pp. 111–23.

14. Flavell, J. H., Green, F. L. & Flavell, E. R., 'Development of children's awareness of their own thoughts', *Journal of Cognition and Development*, 1(1), 2000, pp. 97–112.

15. Herrington, C. G., 'Children's metacognitive development and learning cognitive behavior therapy', PhD dissertation, Vanderbilt University, Tennessee, 2014.

16. Flavell, J. H., Green, F. L. & Flavell, E. R., 'The mind has a mind of its own: Developing knowledge about mental uncontrollability', *Cognitive Development*, 13(1), 1998, pp. 127–38.

17. Ibid.

18. Waters, S. F., West, T. V. & Mendes, W. B., 'Stress contagion: Physiological covariation between mothers and infants', *Psychological Science*, 25(4), 2014, pp. 934–42.

19. Oberle, E. & Schonert-Reichl, K. A., 'Stress contagion in the classroom? The link between classroom teacher burnout and morning cortisol in elementary school students', *Social Science & Medicine*, 159, 2016, pp. 30–7.

20. Price, J. S., 'Evolutionary aspects of anxiety disorders', *Dialogues in Clinical Neuroscience*, 5(3), 2003, pp. 223–36.

21. Peterson, C., 'What is positive psychology, and what is it not?', *Psychology Today* (Australia), 2008.

22. Rapee, R. M., 'Anxiety disorders in children and adolescents: Nature, development, treatment and prevention', 2012.

## Chapter 2

1. Gottschalk, M. G. & Domschke, K., 'Genetics of generalized anxiety disorder and related traits', *Dialogues in Clinical Neuroscience*, 19(2), 2017, pp. 159–68.

2. Holt, M. K. & Espalage, D. L., 'Perceived social support among bullies, victims, and bully-victims', *Journal of Youth and Adolescence*, 36(8), 2007, pp. 984–94.

3.  Platt, R., Williams, S. R. & Ginsburg, G. S., 'Stressful life events and child anxiety: Examining parent and child mediators', *Child Psychiatry and Human Development*, 47(1), 2016, pp. 23–34.

4.  Fremont, W. P., Pataki, C. & Beresin, E. V., 'The impact of terrorism on children and adolescents: Terror in the skies, terror on television', *Child and Adolescent Psychiatric Clinics of North America*, 14(3), 2005, pp. viii, 429–51.

5.  Kar, N. & Bastia, B. K., 'Post-traumatic stress disorder, depression and generalised anxiety disorder in adolescents after a natural disaster: A study of comorbidity', *Clinical Practice and Epidemiology in Mental Health*, 2(17), 2006.

6.  Twenge, J. M., *iGen* (Atria Books: New York), 2017.

7.  Australian Communications and Media Authority, 'Communications report 2011–12 series, Report 3 – Smartphones and tablets take-up and use in Australia', 2013, p. 2.

8.  Twenge, J. M., Martin, G. N. & Campbell, W. K., 'Decreases in psychological well-being among American adolescents after 2012 and links to screen time during the rise of smartphone technology', *Emotion*, 18(6), 2018, pp. 765–80; Zhao, J., Zhang, Y., Jiang, F., Ip, P., Ho, F. K. W., Zhang, Y. & Huang, H., 'Excessive screen time and psychosocial well-being: The mediating role of body mass index, sleep duration, and parent-child interaction', *The Journal of Pediatrics*, 202, 2018, pp. 157–62.

9.  Robinson, T. N., Banda, J. A., Hale, L., Lu, A. S., Fleming-Milici, F., Calvert, S. L. & Wartella, E., 'Screen media exposure and obesity in children and adolescents', *Pediatrics*, 140(Suppl 2), 2017, pp. 97–101.

10. Oh, J. H., Yoo, H., Park, H. K. & Do, Y. R., 'Analysis of circadian properties and healthy levels of blue light from smartphones at night', *Scientific Reports*, 5(1), 2015, p. 11325.

11. Wahlstrom, K., 'Sleepy teenage brains need school to start later in the morning', *The Conversation*, 13 September 2017.

12. De Berardis, D., Marini, S., Fornaro, M., Srinivasan, V., Iasevoli, F., Tomasetti, C., Valchera, A., Perna, G., Quera-Salva, M. A., Martinotti, G. & di Giannantonio, M., 'The melatonergic system in mood and anxiety disorders and the role of agomelatine: Implications for clinical practice', *International Journal of Molecular Sciences*, 14(6), 2013, pp. 12458–83; Malhotra, S., Sawhney, G. & Pandhi, P., 'The therapeutic potential of melatonin: A review of the science', *MedGenMed: Medscape General Medicine*, 6(2), 2004, p. 46; Ochoa-Sanchez, R., Rainer, Q., Comai, S., Spadoni, G., Bedini, A., Rivara, S., Fraschini, F., Mor, M., Tarzia, G. & Gobbi, G., 'Anxiolytic effects of the melatonin MT2 receptor partial agonist UCM765: Comparison with melatonin and diazepam', *Progress in Neuro-Psychopharmacology and Biological Psychiatry*, 39(2), 2012, pp. 318–25.

13. Lambert, G. W., Reid, C., Kaye, D. M., Jennings, G. L., & Esler, M. D., 'Effect of sunlight and season on serotonin turnover in the brain', *The Lancet*, *360*(9348), 2002, pp. 1840–2.

14. Mead, M. N., 'Benefits of sunlight: A bright spot for human health', *Environmental Health Perspectives*, *116*(4), 2008, pp. 160–7.

15. Wurtman, J. J., 'Dropping serotonin levels: Why you crave carbs late in the day', *Huffington Post*, 16 February 2011.

16. Zohar, J. & Westenberg, H. G., 'Anxiety disorders: A review of tricyclic antidepressants and selective serotonin reuptake inhibitors', *Acta Psychiatrica Scandinavica. Supplementum*, *403*, 2000, pp. 39–49.

17. Yoo, S.-S., Gujar, N., Hu, P., Jolesz, F. A. & Walker, M. P., 'The human emotional brain without sleep – a prefrontal amygdala disconnect', *Current Biology*, *17*(20), 2007, pp. 877–8.

18. Haynes, T. & Clements, R., 'Dopamine, smartphones & you: A battle for your time', *Science in the News* blog, Harvard University Graduate School of Arts and Sciences, 1 May 2018.

19. Twenge, J. M., 'Have Smartphones Destroyed a Generation?', *The Atlantic*, September 2017.

20. Common Sense Media, 'The Common Sense census: Media use by tweens and teens', 2015.

21. Fahy, A. E., Stansfeld, S. A., Smuk, M., Smith, N. R., Cummins, S. & Clark, C., 'Longitudinal associations between cyberbullying involvement and adolescent mental health', *Journal of Adolescent Health*, *59*(5), 2016, pp. 502–9.

22. Beyond Blue, 'Bullying and cyberbullying'.

23. Visit www.ditchthelabel.org for the largest anti-bullying support hub in the world.

24. Spence, n.d.; moodgym cognitive behavioural therapy training program, n.d.; Grose & Richardson.

25. Rothman, L., 'The computer in society: Sorry, this 50-year-old prediction is wrong', *Time*, 2 April 2015.

26. OECD, *How's Life? 2017: Measuring well-being*, OECD Publishing, 2017.

27. Dinh, H., Strazdins, L. & Welsh, J., 'Hour-glass ceilings: Work-hour thresholds, gendered health inequities', *Social Science & Medicine*, *176*, 2017, pp. 42–51.

28. Strazdins, L., OBrien, L. V., Lucas, N. & Rodgers, B., 'Combining work and family: Rewards or risks for children's mental health?', *Social Science & Medicine*, *87*, 2013, pp. 99–107.

29. McLoyd, V. C., 'The impact of economic hardship on Black families and children: Psychological distress, parenting, and socioemotional development', *Child Development*, *61*(2), 1990, pp. 311–46.

30. Gray, P., 'The decline of play and the rise of psychopathology in children and adolescents', *American Journal of Play*, *3*(4), 2011, pp. 443–63.

## Chapter 3

1.  Shin, L. M. & Liberzon, I., 'The neurocircuitry of fear, stress, and anxiety disorders', *Neuropsychopharmacology: Official publication of the American College of Neuropsychopharmacology*, 35(1), 2010, pp. 169–91.
2.  Qin, S., Young, C. B., Duan, X., Chen, T., Supekar, K. & Menon, V., 'Amygdala subregional structure and intrinsic functional connectivity predicts individual differences in anxiety during early childhood', *Biological Psychiatry*, 75(11), 2014, pp. 892–900.
3.  Bishop, S., Duncan, J., Brett, M. & Lawrence, A. D., 'Prefrontal cortical function and anxiety: Controlling attention to threat-related stimuli', *Nature Neuroscience*, 7(2), 2004, pp. 184–8; Park, J., Wood, J., Bondi, C., Del Arco, A. & Moghaddam, B., 'Anxiety evokes hypofrontality and disrupts rule-relevant encoding by dorsomedial prefrontal cortex neurons', *Journal of Neuroscience: The official journal of the Society for Neuroscience*, 36(11), 2016, pp. 3322–35.
4.  Leung, M.-K., Lau, W. K. W., Chan, C. C. H., Wong, S. S. Y., Fung, A. L. C. & Lee, T. M. C., 'Meditation-induced neuroplastic changes in amygdala activity during negative affective processing', *Social Neuroscience*, 13(3), 2018, pp. 277–88; Taren, A. A., Creswell, J. D. & Gianaros, P. J., 'Dispositional mindfulness co-varies with smaller amygdala and caudate volumes in community adults', *PLoS ONE*, 8(5), 2013, e64574.
5.  Harvard Health Publishing, 'Understanding the stress response', March 2011.

## Chapter 4

1.  Merikangas, K. R., He, J.-P., Burstein, M., Swanson, S. A., Avenevoli, S., Cui, L., Benjet, C., Georgiades, K. & Swendsen, J., 'Lifetime prevalence of mental disorders in U.S. adolescents: Results from the National Comorbidity Survey Replication – Adolescent Supplement (NCS-A)', *Journal of the American Academy of Child and Adolescent Psychiatry*, 49(10), 2010, pp. 980–9.
2.  Kessler, R. C., Amminger, G. P., Aguilar-Gaxiola, S., Alonso, J., Lee, S. & Üstün, T. B., 'Age of onset of mental disorders: A review of recent literature', *Current Opinion in Psychiatry*, 20(4), 2007, pp. 359–64.
3.  Siddaway, A. P., Taylor, P. J. & Wood, A. M., 'Reconceptualizing anxiety as a continuum that ranges from high calmness to high anxiety: The joint importance of reducing distress and increasing well-being', *Journal of Personality and Social Psychology*, 114(2), 2018, pp. e1–e11.
4.  Miller, L., *The silent epidemic: Anxiety disorders in school children*, 2012.
5.  Beesdo, K., Knappe, S. & Pine, D. S., 'Anxiety and anxiety disorders in children and adolescents: Developmental issues and implications for DSM-V', *Psychiatric Clinics of North America*, 32(3), 2009, pp. 483–524; Young, K., 'Fear and anxiety – An age by age guide to common fears, the reasons for each and how to manage them', *Hey Sigmund*, n.d.

6. Beesdo, Knappe & Pine, 2009.
7. Beyond Blue, 'A parents' guide to anxiety and depression in young people', n.d..
8. Beyond Blue, 'Anxiety in Children', n.d.; Anxiety Canada, 'Managing an anxious child – where to start', 2017; Rapee, 2012.
9. Beyond Blue, 'Anxiety in Children', n.d.
10. Rapee, 2012.
11. Crome, E., Grove, R., Baillie, A. J., Sunderland, M., Teesson, M. & Slade, T., 'DSM-IV and DSM-5 social anxiety disorder in the Australian community', *Australian and New Zealand Journal of Psychiatry, 49*(3), 2015, pp. 227–35.
12. American Psychiatric Association, *Diagnostic and Statistical Manual of Mental Disorders, 5th Edition* (APA: Arlington, VA), 2013.
13. Canadian Mental Health Association, 'Anxiety Disorders in Children and Youth', *Visions, 14*(Spring), 2002.
14. Boileau, B., 'A review of obsessive-compulsive disorder in children and adolescents', *Dialogues in Clinical Neuroscience, 13*(4), 2011, pp. 401–11.
15. Geller, D. A., 'Obsessive-compulsive and spectrum disorders in children and adolescents', *Psychiatric Clinics of North America, 29*(2), 2006, pp. 353–70.

## Chapter 6

1. McCurry, C., *Working with Parents of Anxious Children: Therapeutic strategies for encouraging communication, coping, and change* (W. W. Norton & Company: New York), 2015.

## Chapter 7

1. Witt, S., *Raising Resilient Kids* (Collective Wisdom Publications: Melbourne) 2018, p. 5.

## Chapter 9

1. 'Checking in' information from Brackett, M., Ruler Program, n.d.

## Chapter 10

1. Goldman, B., 'Study shows how slow breathing induces tranquility', Stanford Medicine News Center, 30 March 2017.

## Chapter 14

1. Cooper, L., 'Australia, we have a sleep deprivation problem', *Huffington Post*, 7 February 2017.

## Chapter 16

1. Brown, B., 'Why goofing off is really good for you', *Huffington Post*, 3 February 2014.

2. Alexander, J. J. & Sandahl, I., *The Danish Way of Parenting: What the happiest people in the world know about raising confident, capable kids* (TarcherPerigee: New York), 2016, p. 16.
3. Sutton-Smith, B., 'We study play because life is hard', *Psychology Today* (Australia), 2015.
4. Lazarus, R. S., Dodd, H. F., Majdandžić, M., de Vente, W., Morris, T., Byrow, Y., Bögels, S. M. & Hudson, J. L., 'The relationship between challenging parenting behaviour and childhood anxiety disorders', *Journal of Affective Disorders, 190*, 2016, pp. 784–91.

## Chapter 17

1. Kennedy, R., 'Children spend half the time playing outside in comparison to their parents', *Child in the City*, 15 January 2018.
2. www.parentingideas.com.au/schools/insight/role-parents-screen-time/ (only members can access this article)
3. Twohig-Bennett, C. & Jones, A., 'The health benefits of the great outdoors: A systematic review and meta-analysis of greenspace exposure and health outcomes', *Environmental Research, 166*, 2018, pp. 628–37.

## Chapter 18

1. Harris, R., *The Happiness Trap: Stop struggling, start living* (Exisle Publishing: Wollombi, NSW), 2007, p. 169.
2. Ibid., p. 171.
3. Some of these are included in our Parenting Anxious Kids online course available at www.parentingideas.com.au/product/parenting-anxious-kids-online-course.

## Chapter 19

1. Australian Bureau of Statistics, 'General Social Survey: Summary Results, Australia, 2014', 2015.

## Chapter 20

1. Benard, B., *Resiliency: What we have learned* (WestEd: San Francisco), 2004, p. 10.

## Chapter 21

1. Australian Government Department of Health, 'Better access to mental health care: Fact sheet for patients', n.d.
2. Ungar, M. P. D., 'Finding a great therapist for your child', *Psychology Today*, 5 November 2010.

## Chapter 22

1. James, A. C., James, G., Cowdrey, F. A., Soler, A. & Choke, A., 'Cognitive behavioural therapy for anxiety disorders in children and adolescents', *Cochrane Database of Systematic Reviews* (2), 2015.

2. Beck, J. S., *Cognitive Behavior Therapy: Basics and beyond*, 2nd Edition (Guilford Press: New York), 2011.
3. 'Examples of fear ladders' adapted from Anxiety Canada, n.d.
4. Ipser, J. C., Stein, D. J., Hawkridge, S. & Hoppe, L., 'Pharmacotherapy for anxiety disorders in children and adolescents', *Cochrane Database of Systematic Reviews* (3), 2009.
5. Creswell, C., Waite, P. & Cooper, P. J., 'Assessment and management of anxiety disorders in children and adolescents', *Archives of Disease in Childhood*, 99(7), 2014, pp. 674–8.
6. Eifert, G. H. & Forsyth, J. P., *Acceptance & Commitment Therapy for Anxiety Disorders: A practitioner's treatment guide to using mindfulness, acceptance, and values-based behavior change strategies* (New Harbinger Publications: Oakland, CA), 2005.
7. Ibid.
8. Ibid.

## Chapter 23

1. Asthana, A. & Boycott-Owen, M., '"Epidemic of stress" blamed for 3,750 teachers on long-term sick leave', *The Guardian*, 11 January 2018.
2. Walker, T., 'How many teachers are highly stressed? Maybe more than people think', neaToday, 11 May 2018.

# Bibliography

Alexander, J. J. & Sandahl, I. (2016). *The Danish Way of Parenting: What the happiest people in the world know about raising confident, capable kids.* TarcherPerigee, New York.

American Psychiatric Association (2013). *Diagnostic and Statistical Manual of Mental Disorders,* 5th Edition, APA, Arlington, VA.

Anxiety Canada (2017). 'Managing an anxious child – where to start'. Retrieved 7 March 2019 from www.anxietycanada.com/resources/blog/managing-anxious-child---where-start

—— (n.d.). 'Examples of fear ladders'. Retrieved 7 March 2019 from www.anxietycanada.com/sites/default/files/Examples_of_Fear_Ladders.pdf

Asthana, A. & Boycott-Owen, M. (2018). '"Epidemic of stress" blamed for 3,750 teachers on long-term sick leave', *The Guardian.* Retrieved 6 March 2019 from www.theguardian.com/education/2018/jan/11/epidemic-of-stress-blamed-for-3750-teachers-on-longterm-sick-leave

Australian Bureau of Statistics (2015). 'General Social Survey: Summary Results, Australia, 2014'. Retrieved 7 March 2019 from www.abs.gov.au/ausstats/abs@.nsf/Latestproducts/4159.0Main%20Features152014

Australian Communications and Media Authority (2013). 'Communications report 2011–12 series, Report 3 – Smartphones and tablets: Take-up and use in Australia', see also www.acma.gov.au/theACMA/Library/researchacma/Research-reports/smartphone-use-soars

Australian Government Department of Health (n.d.). 'Better access to mental health care: Fact sheet for patients'. Retrieved 7 March 2019 from www.health.gov.au/internet/main/publishing.nsf/content/mental-ba-fact-pat

Australian Institute of Health and Welfare (2018). 'Australia's Health 2018: In brief'. Retrieved 7 March 2019 from www.aihw.gov.au/getmedia/fe037cf1-0cd0-4663-a8c0-67cd09b1f30c/aihw-aus-222.pdf.aspx

Beck, J. S. (2011). *Cognitive Behavior Therapy: Basics and beyond, 2nd Edition.* Guilford Press, New York.

Beesdo, K., Knappe, S. & Pine, D. S. (2009). 'Anxiety and anxiety disorders in children and adolescents: Developmental issues and implications for DSM-V', *Psychiatric Clinics of North America, 32*(3), pp. 483–524. Retrieved 7 March 2019 from https://doi.org/10.1016/j.psc.2009.06.002

Benard, B. (2004). *Resiliency: What we have learned.* WestEd, San Francisco.

Beyond Blue (n.d.). 'A parent's guide to anxiety and depression in young people'. Retrieved 7 March 2019 from http://resources.beyondblue.org.au/prism/file?token=BL/1061

—— (n.d.). 'Bullying and cyberbullying'. Retrieved 13 September 2018, from www.youthbeyondblue.com/understand-what's-going-on/bullying-and-cyberbullying

—— (n.d.). 'Anxiety in children'. Retrieved 2 October 2018, from https://healthyfamilies.beyondblue.org.au/age-6-12/mental-health-conditions-in-children/anxiety

Bhatia, M. S. & Goyal, A. (2018). 'Anxiety disorders in children and adolescents: Need for early detection', *Journal of Postgraduate Medicine, 64*(2), pp. 75–6. Retrieved 7 March 2019 from https://doi.org/10.4103/jpgm.JPGM_65_18

Bishop, S., Duncan, J., Brett, M. & Lawrence, A. D. (2004). 'Prefrontal cortical function and anxiety: Controlling attention to threat-related stimuli', *Nature Neuroscience, 7*(2), pp. 184–8. Retrieved 7 March 2019 from https://doi.org/10.1038/nn1173

Boileau, B. (2011). 'A review of obsessive-compulsive disorder in children and adolescents', *Dialogues in Clinical Neuroscience, 13*(4), pp. 401–11. Retrieved 7 March 2019 from www.ncbi.nlm.nih.gov/pubmed/22275846

Brackett, M. (n.d.). Ruler Program, Yale Center for Emotional Intelligence. Retrieved 7 March 2019 from http://ei.yale.edu/ruler

Brown, A. M., Deacon, B. J., Abramowitz, J. S., Dammann, J. & Whiteside, S. P. (2007). 'Parents' perceptions of pharmacological and cognitive-behavioral treatments for childhood anxiety disorders', *Behaviour Research and Therapy, 45*(4), pp. 819–28. Retrieved 7 March 2019 from https://doi.org/10.1016/j.brat.2006.04.010

Brown, B. (2014). 'Why goofing off is really good for you', *Huffington Post.* Retrieved 7 March 2019 from www.huffingtonpost.com/2014/02/03/brene-brown-importance-of-play_n_4675625.html

Canadian Mental Health Association (2002). 'Anxiety Disorders in Children and Youth', *Visions, 14*(Spring). Retrieved 7 March 2019 from https://cmha.bc.ca/wp-content/uploads/2016/07/visions_anxietyCY.pdf

Common Sense Media (2015). 'The Common Sense census: Media use by tweens and teens'. Retrieved 7 March from www.commonsensemedia.org/sites/default/files/uploads/research/census_researchreport.pdf

Cooper, L. (2017). 'Australia, we have a sleep deprivation problem', *Huffington Post*. Retrieved 7 March 2019 from www.huffingtonpost.com.au/2017/02/07/australia-we-have-a-sleep-deprivation-problem_a_21708513/

Creswell, C., Waite, P. & Cooper, P. J. (2014). 'Assessment and management of anxiety disorders in children and adolescents', *Archives of Disease in Childhood, 99*(7), pp. 674–8. Retrieved 7 March 2019 from https://doi.org/10.1136/archdischild-2013-303768

Crome, E., Grove, R., Baillie, A. J., Sunderland, M., Teesson, M. & Slade, T. (2015). 'DSM-IV and DSM-5 social anxiety disorder in the Australian community', *Australian and New Zealand Journal of Psychiatry, 49*(3), pp. 227–35. Retrieved 7 March 2019 from https://doi.org/10.1177/0004867414546699

De Berardis, D., Marini, S., Fornaro, M., Srinivasan, V., Iasevoli, F., Tomasetti, C., Valchera, A., Perna, G., Quera-Salva, M. A., Martinotti, G., di Giannantonio, M. (2013). 'The melatonergic system in mood and anxiety disorders and the role of agomelatine: Implications for clinical practice', *International Journal of Molecular Sciences, 14*(6), pp. 12458–83. Retrieved 7 March 2019 from https://doi.org/10.3390/ijms140612458

Dinh, H., Strazdins, L. & Welsh, J. (2017). 'Hour-glass ceilings: Work-hour thresholds, gendered health inequities', *Social Science & Medicine, 176*, pp. 42–51. Retrieved 7 March 2019 from https://doi.org/10.1016/J.SOCSCIMED.2017.01.024

Ditch the Label (2017). 'The Annual Bullying survey 2017'. Retrieved 7 March 2019 from www.ditchthelabel.org/wp-content/uploads/2017/07/The-Annual-Bullying-Survey-2017-1.pdf

Eifert, G. H. & Forsyth, J. P. (2005). *Acceptance & Commitment Therapy for Anxiety Disorders: A practitioner's treatment guide to using mindfulness, acceptance, and values-based behavior change strategies.* New Harbinger Publications, Oakland.

Fahy, A. E., Stansfeld, S. A., Smuk, M., Smith, N. R., Cummins, S. & Clark, C. (2016). 'Longitudinal associations between cyberbullying involvement and adolescent mental health', *Journal of Adolescent Health, 59*(5), pp. 502–9. Retrieved 7 March 2019 from https://doi.org/10.1016/j.jadohealth.2016.06.006

Flavell, J. H., Green, F. L. & Flavell, E. R. (1998). 'The mind has a mind of its own: Developing knowledge about mental uncontrollability', *Cognitive Development, 13*(1), pp. 127–38. Retrieved 7 March 2019 from https://doi.org/10.1016/S0885-2014(98)90024-7

—— (2000). 'Development of children's awareness of their own thoughts', *Journal of Cognition and Development, 1*(1), pp. 97–112. Retrieved 7 March 2019 from https://doi.org/10.1207/S15327647JCD0101N_10

Fremont, W. P., Pataki, C., & Beresin, E. V. (2005). 'The impact of terrorism on children and adolescents: Terror in the skies, terror on television', *Child and Adolescent Psychiatric Clinics of North America, 14*(3), pp. viii, 429–51. Retrieved 7 March 2019 from https://doi.org/10.1016/j.chc.2005.02.001

Geller, D. A. (2006). 'Obsessive-compulsive and spectrum disorders in children and adolescents', *Psychiatric Clinics of North America, 29*(2), pp. 353–70. Retrieved 7 March 2019 from https://doi.org/10.1016/j.psc.2006.02.012

Goldman, B. (2017). 'Study shows how slow breathing induces tranquility', Stanford Medicine News Center. Retrieved 7 March 2019 from www.med.stanford.edu/news/all-news/2017/03/study-discovers-how-slow-breathing-induces-tranquility.html

Gottschalk, M. G. & Domschke, K. (2017). 'Genetics of generalized anxiety disorder and related traits', *Dialogues in Clinical Neuroscience, 19*(2), pp. 159–68. Retrieved 7 March 2019 from www.ncbi.nlm.nih.gov/pubmed/28867940

Gray, P. (2011). 'The decline of play and the rise of psychopathology in children and adolescents', *Americal Journal of Play, 3*(4), pp. 443–63. Retrieved 7 March 2019 from www.researchgate.net/publication/265449180_The_Decline_of_Play_and_the_Rise_of_Psychopathology_in_Children_and_Adolescents

Gregory, A. M., Caspi, A., Moffitt, T. E., Koenen, K, Eley, T. C. & Poulton, R. (2007). 'Juvenile mental health histories of adults with anxiety disorders', *American Journal of Psychiatry, 164*(2), pp. 301–8. Retrieved 7 March 2019 from https://ajp.psychiatryonline.org/doi/pdfplus/10.1176/ajp.2007.164.2.301

Grose, M. & Richardson, J. (n.d.). 'Parenting anxious kids online course'. Retrieved 7 March 2019 from www.parentingideas.com.au/product/parenting-anxious-kids-online-course/

Harris, R. (2007). *The Happiness Trap: Stop struggling, start living.* Exisle Publishing, Wollombi, NSW.

Harvard Health Publishing (2011). 'Understanding the stress response'. Retrieved 7 March 2019 from www.health.harvard.edu/staying-healthy/understanding-the-stress-response

Haynes, T. & Clements, R. (2018). 'Dopamine, smartphones & you: A battle for your time', *Science in the News* blog, Harvard University Graduate School of Arts and Sciences. Retrieved 6 March 2019 from http://sitn.hms.harvard.edu/flash/2018/dopamine-smartphones-battle-time/

Herrington, C. G. (2014). 'Children's metacognitive development and learning cognitive behavior therapy', PhD dissertation, Vanderbilt University, Tennessee. Retrieved 7 March 2019 from https://etd.library.vanderbilt.edu/available/etd-07252014-181342/unrestricted/herrington.pdf

Hiscock, H., Neely, R. J., Lei, S. & Freed, G. (2018). 'Paediatric mental and physical health presentations to emergency departments, Victoria, 2008–15', *Medical Journal of Australia, 208*(8), pp. 343–8. Retrieved 7 March 2019 from https://doi.org/10.5694/mja17.00434

Holt, M. K. & Espalage, D. L. (2007). 'Perceived social support among bullies, victims, and bully-victims', *Journal of Youth and Adolescence, 36*(8), pp. 984–94. Retrieved 7 March 2019 from https://doi.org/10.5694/mja17.00434

Ialongo, N., Edelsohn, G., Werthamer-Larsson, L., Crockett, L. & Kellam, S. (1994). 'The significance of self-reported anxious symptoms in first-grade children', *Journal of Abnormal Child Psychology*, 22(4), pp. 441–55. Retrieved 7 March 2019 from www.ncbi.nlm.nih.gov/pubmed/7963077

Ipser, J. C., Stein, D. J., Hawkridge, S. & Hoppe, L. (2009). 'Pharmacotherapy for anxiety disorders in children and adolescents', *Cochrane Database of Systematic Reviews* (3). Retrieved 7 March 2019 from https://doi.org/10.1002/14651858.CD005170.pub2

James, A. C., James, G., Cowdrey, F. A., Soler, A., & Choke, A. (2015). 'Cognitive behavioural therapy for anxiety disorders in children and adolescents', *Cochrane Database of Systematic Reviews* (2). Retrieved 7 March 2019 from https://doi.org/10.1002/14651858.CD004690.pub4

Kar, N. & Bastia, B. K. (2006). 'Post-traumatic stress disorder, depression and generalised anxiety disorder in adolescents after a natural disaster: A study of comorbidity', *Clinical Practice and Epidemiology in Mental Health*, 2(17). Retrieved 7 March 2019 from https://doi.org/10.1186/1745-0179-2-17

Kennedy, R. (2018). 'Children spend half the time playing outside in comparison to their parents', *Child in the City*. Retrieved 7 March 2019 from www.childinthecity.org/2018/01/15/children-spend-half-the-time-playing-outside-in-comparison-to-their-parents/

Kessler, R. C., Amminger, G. P., Aguilar-Gaxiola, S., Alonso, J., Lee, S. & Üstün, T. B. (2007). 'Age of onset of mental disorders: A review of recent literature', *Current Opinion in Psychiatry*, 20(4), pp. 359–64. Retrieved 7 March 2019 from https://doi.org/10.1097/YCO.0b013e32816ebc8c

Kessler, R. C., Berglund, P., Demler, O., Jin, R., Merikangas, K. R. & Walters, E. E. (2005). 'Lifetime prevalence and age-of-onset distributions of DSM-IV disorders in the National Comorbidity Survey Replication', *Archives of General Psychiatry*, 62(6), p. 593. Retrieved 7 March 2019 from https://doi.org/10.1001/archpsyc.62.6.593

Lambert, G. W., Reid, C., Kaye, D. M., Jennings, G. L. & Esler, M. D. (2002). 'Effect of sunlight and season on serotonin turnover in the brain', *The Lancet*, 360(9348), pp. 1840–2. Retrieved 7 March 2019 from www.ncbi.nlm.nih.gov/pubmed/12480364

Lazarus, R. S., Dodd, H. F., Majdandžić, M., de Vente, W., Morris, T., Byrow, Y., Bögels, S. M. & Hudson, J. L. (2016). 'The relationship between challenging parenting behaviour and childhood anxiety disorders', *Journal of Affective Disorders*, 190, pp. 784–91. Retrieved 7 March 2019 from https://doi.org/10.1016/J.JAD.2015.11.032

Leung, M.-K., Lau, W. K. W., Chan, C. C. H., Wong, S. S. Y., Fung, A. L. C. & Lee, T. M. C. (2018). 'Meditation-induced neuroplastic changes in amygdala activity during negative affective processing', *Social Neuroscience*, 13(3), pp. 277–288. Retrieved 7 March 2019 from https://doi.org/10.1080/17470919.2017.1311939

Leutwyler, B. (2009). 'Metacognitive learning strategies: Differential development patterns in high school', *Metacognition and Learning*, 4(2), pp. 111–23. Retrieved 7 March 2019 from https://doi.org/10.1007/s11409-009-9037-5

Malhotra, S., Sawhney, G. & Pandhi, P. (2004). 'The therapeutic potential of melatonin: A review of the science', *MedGenMed: Medscape General Medicine*, 6(2), p. 46. Retrieved 7 March 2019 from www.ncbi.nlm.nih.gov/pubmed/15266271

McCurry, C. (2015). *Working with Parents of Anxious Children: Therapeutic strategies for encouraging communcation, coping, and change.* W. W. Norton & Company, New York

McLoyd, V. C. (1990). 'The impact of economic hardship on Black families and children: Psychological distress, parenting, and socioemotional development', *Child Development*, 61(2), pp. 311–46. Retrieved 7 March 2019 from www.ncbi.nlm.nih.gov/pubmed/2188806

Mead, M. N. (2008). 'Benefits of sunlight: A bright spot for human health', *Environmental Health Perspectives*, 116(4), pp. 160–7. Retrieved 7 March 2019 from https://doi.org/10.1289/ehp.116-a160

Merikangas, K. R., He, J.-P., Burstein, M., Swanson, S. A., Avenevoli, S., Cui, L., Benjet, C., Georgiades, K. & Swendsen, J. (2010). 'Lifetime prevalence of mental disorders in U.S. adolescents: Results from the National Comorbidity Survey Replication – Adolescent Supplement (NCS-A)', *Journal of the American Academy of Child and Adolescent Psychiatry*, 49(10), pp. 980–9. Retrieved 7 March 2019 from https://doi.org/10.1016/j.jaac.2010.05.017

Miller, L. (2012). *The silent epidemic: Anxiety disorders in school children.* Retrieved 6 March 2019 from https://news.ubc.ca/2012/04/16/early-screening-for-anxiety-disorders-in-children-helps-prevent-mental-health-concerns-ubc-study. No longer available

National Society for the Prevention of Cruelty to Children (2016). 'Anxiety a rising concern in young people contacting Childline'. Retrieved 7 March 2019 from www.nspcc.org.uk/what-we-do/news-opinion/anxiety-rising-concern-young-people-contacting-childline/

Oberle, E. & Schonert-Reichl, K. A. (2016). 'Stress contagion in the classroom? The link between classroom teacher burnout and morning cortisol in elementary school students', *Social Science & Medicine*, 159, pp. 30–37. Retrieved 7 March 2019 from https://doi.org/10.1016/J.SOCSCIMED.2016.04.031

Ochoa-Sanchez, R., Rainer, Q., Comai, S., Spadoni, G., Bedini, A., Rivara, S., Fraschini, F., Mor, M., Tarzia, G. & Gobbi, G. (2012). 'Anxiolytic effects of the melatonin MT2 receptor partial agonist UCM765: Comparison with melatonin and diazepam', *Progress in Neuro-Psychopharmacology and Biological Psychiatry*, 39(2), pp. 318–25. Retrieved 7 March 2019 from https://doi.org/10.1016/j.pnpbp.2012.07.003

OECD (2017). *How's Life? 2017: Measuring Well-being*, OECD Publishing. Retrieved 7 March 2019 from https://doi.org/10.1787/how_life-2017-en

Oh, J. H., Yoo, H., Park, H. K., & Do, Y. R. (2015). 'Analysis of circadian properties and healthy levels of blue light from smartphones at night', *Scientific Reports*, 5(1), p. 11325. Retrieved 7 March 2019 from https://doi.org/10.1038/srep11325

Park, J., Wood, J., Bondi, C., Del Arco, A. & Moghaddam, B. (2016). 'Anxiety evokes hypofrontality and disrupts rule-relevant encoding by dorsomedial prefrontal cortex neurons', *Journal of Neuroscience: The official journal of the Society for Neuroscience*, 36(11), pp. 3322–35. Retrieved 7 March 2019 from https://doi.org/10.1523/JNEUROSCI.4250-15.2016

Peterson, C. (2008). 'What is positive psychology, and what is it not?', *Psychology Today* (Australia). Retrieved 6 March 2019 from www.psychologytoday.com/au/blog/the-good-life/200805/what-is-positive-psychology-and-what-is-it-not

Platt, R., Williams, S. R., & Ginsburg, G. S. (2016). 'Stressful life events and child anxiety: Examining parent and child mediators', *Child Psychiatry and Human Development*, 47(1), pp. 23–34. Retrieved 7 March 2019 from https://doi.org/10.1007/s10578-015-0540-4

Polanczyk, G. V., Salum, G. A., Sugaya, L. S., Caye, A. & Rohde, L. A. (2015). 'Annual research review: A meta-analysis of the worldwide prevalence of mental disorders in children and adolescents', *Journal of Child Psychology and Psychiatry*, 56(3), pp. 345–65. Retrieved 7 March 2019 from https://doi.org/10.1111/jcpp.12381

Price, J. S. (2003). 'Evolutionary aspects of anxiety disorders', *Dialogues in Clinical Neuroscience*, 5(3), pp. 223–36. Retrieved 7 March 2019 from www.ncbi.nlm.nih.gov/pubmed/22033473

Qin, S., Young, C. B., Duan, X., Chen, T., Supekar, K. & Menon, V. (2014). 'Amygdala subregional structure and intrinsic functional connectivity predicts individual differences in anxiety during early childhood', *Biological Psychiatry*, 75(11), pp. 892–900. Retrieved 7 March 2019 from https://doi.org/10.1016/j.biopsych.2013.10.006

Rapee, R. M. (2012). 'Anxiety disorders in children and adolescents: Nature, development, treatment and prevention', in Rey, J. M. (ed.), *IACAPAP e-Textbook of Child and Adolescent Mental Health*. International Association for Child and Adolescent Psychiatry and Allied Professions, Geneva, pp. 1–19. Retrieved 7 March 2019 from http://iacapap.org/wp-content/uploads/F.1-ANXIETY-DISORDERS-072012.pdf

Robinson, T. N., Banda, J. A., Hale, L., Lu, A. S., Fleming-Milici, F., Calvert, S. L. & Wartella, E. (2017). 'Screen media exposure and obesity in children and adolescents', *Pediatrics*, 140(Suppl 2), pp. 97–101. Retrieved 7 March 2019 from https://doi.org/10.1542/peds.2016-1758K

Rothman, L. (2015). 'The computer in society: Sorry, this 50-Year-old prediction is wrong', *Time*. Retrieved 7 March 2019 from http://time.com/3754781/1965-predictions-computers/

Shin, L. M., & Liberzon, I. (2010). 'The neurocircuitry of fear, stress, and anxiety disorders', *Neuropsychopharmacology: Official publication of the American College of Neuropsychopharmacology, 35*(1), pp. 169–91. Retrieved 7 March 2019 from https://doi.org/10.1038/npp.2009.83

Siddaway, A. P., Taylor, P. J., & Wood, A. M. (2018). 'Reconceptualizing anxiety as a continuum that ranges from high calmness to high anxiety: The joint importance of reducing distress and increasing well-being', *Journal of Personality and Social Psychology, 114*(2), pp. e1–e11. Retrieved 7 March 2019 from https://doi.org/10.1037/pspp0000128

Spence, S. (n.d.). 'BRAVE-Online: Helping young people overcome anxiety'. Retrieved 7 March 2019 from www.brave-online.com

Strazdins, L., OBrien, L. V., Lucas, N., & Rodgers, B. (2013). 'Combining work and family: Rewards or risks for children's mental health?', *Social Science & Medicine, 87*, pp. 99–107. Retrieved 7 March 2019 from https://doi.org/10.1016/j.socscimed.2013.03.030

Sutton-Smith, B. (2015). 'We study play because life is hard', *Psychology Today* (Australia). Retrieved 6 March 2019 from https://www.psychologytoday.com/au/blog/having-fun/201509/we-study-play-because-life-is-hard

Taren, A. A., Creswell, J. D., & Gianaros, P. J. (2013). 'Dispositional mindfulness co-varies with smaller amygdala and caudate volumes in community adults', *PLoS ONE, 8*(5), e64574. Retrieved 7 March 2019 from https://doi.org/10.1371/journal.pone.0064574

Twenge, J. M. (2000). 'The age of anxiety? The birth cohort change in anxiety and neuroticism, 1952–1993', *Journal of Personality and Social Psychology, 79*(6), pp. 1007–21. Retrieved 7 March 2019 from http://citeseerx.ist.psu.edu/viewdoc/download?doi=10.1.1.360.8349&rep=rep1&type=pdf

—— (2017). *iGen*. Atria Books, New York

—— (2017). 'Have smartphones destroyed a generation?', *The Atlantic*. Retrieved 7 March 2019 from www.theatlantic.com/magazine/archive/2017/09/has-the-smartphone-destroyed-a-generation/534198/

Twenge, J. M., Gentile, B., Dewall, C. N., Ma, D., Lacefield, K. & Schurtz, D. R. (2010). 'Birth cohort increases in psychopathology among young Americans, 1938–2007: A cross-temporal meta-analysis of the MMPI', *Clinical Psychology Review, 30*(2), pp. 145–54. Retrieved 7 March 2019 from https://doi.org/10.1016/j.cpr.2009.10.005

Twenge, J. M., Martin, G. N., & Campbell, W. K. (2018). 'Decreases in psychological well-being among American adolescents after 2012 and links to screen time during the rise of smartphone technology', *Emotion, 18*(6), pp. 765–80. Retrieved 7 March 2019 from https://doi.org/10.1037/emo0000403

Twohig-Bennett, C. & Jones, A. (2018). 'The health benefits of the great outdoors: A systematic review and meta-analysis of greenspace exposure and health outcomes', *Environmental Research*, 166, pp. 628–37. Retrieved 7 March 2019 from https://doi.org/10.1016/j.envres.2018.06.030

Ungar, M. P. D. (2010). 'Finding a great therapist for your child', *Psychology Today*. Retrieved 6 March 2019 from www.psychologytoday.com/us/blog/nurturing-resilience/201011/finding-great-therapist-your-child

Wahlstrom, K. (2017). 'Sleepy teenage brains need school to start later in the morning', *The Conversation*. Retrieved 7 March 2019 from https://theconversation.com/sleepy-teenage-brains-need-school-to-start-later-in-the-morning-82484

Walker, T. (2018). 'How many teachers are highly stressed? Maybe more than people think', neaToday. Retrieved 6 March 2019 from www.neatoday.org/2018/05/11/study-high-teacher-stress-levels

Waters, S. F., West, T. V, & Mendes, W. B. (2014). 'Stress contagion: Physiological covariation between mothers and infants', *Psychological Science*, 25(4), pp. 934–42. Retrieved 7 March 2019 from https://doi.org/10.1177/0956797613518352

Witt, S. (2018). *Raising Resilient Kids*. Collective Wisdom Publications, Melbourne.

Wurtman, J. J. (2011). 'Dropping serotonin levels: Why you crave carbs late in the day', *Huffington Post*. Retrieved 7 March 2019 from www.huffingtonpost.com/judith-j-wurtman-phd/dropping-serotonin-levels-_b_819855.html

Xin, Z., Zhang, L. & Liu, D. (2010). 'Birth cohort changes of Chinese adolescents' anxiety: A cross-temporal meta-analysis, 1992–2005', *Personality and Individual Differences*, 48(2), pp. 208–12. Retrieved 7 March 2019 from https://doi.org/10.1016/J.PAID.2009.10.010

Yoo, S.-S., Gujar, N., Hu, P., Jolesz, F. A., & Walker, M. P. (2007). 'The human emotional brain without sleep – a prefrontal amygdala disconnect', *Current Biology,* 17(20), pp. 877–8. Retrieved 7 March 2019 from www.sciencedirect.com/science/article/pii/S0960982207017836

Young, K. (n.d.). 'Fear and anxiety – An age by age guide to common fears, the reasons for each and how to manage them', *Hey Sigmund*. Retrieved 7 March 2019 from www.heysigmund.com/age-by-age-guide-to-fears

Young Minds Matter Mental Health Survey (2015). Retrieved 18 June 2018 from https://youngmindsmatter.telethonkids.org.au

Zhao, J., Zhang, Y., Jiang, F., Ip, P., Ho, F. K. W., Zhang, Y. & Huang, H. (2018). 'Excessive screen time and psychosocial well-being: The mediating role of body mass index, sleep duration, and parent-child interaction', *The Journal of Pediatrics*, pp. 157–62. Retrieved 7 March 2019 from https://doi.org/10.1016/j.jpeds.2018.06.029

Zohar, J. & Westenberg, H. G. (2000). 'Anxiety disorders: A review of tricyclic antidepressants and selective serotonin reuptake inhibitors', *Acta Psychiatrica Scandinavica. Supplementum, 403*, pp. 39–49. Retrieved 7 March 2019 from www.ncbi.nlm.nih.gov/pubmed/11019934

# Acknowledgements

*Anxious Kids* is the book we were meant to write together. Each of us has experienced anxiety. Both of us have parented anxious kids and were raised by parents who didn't know what anxiety was, nor what to do about it. Our sincere hope is that this book supports anxious children all over the world to learn to manage their anxiety and thrive, with their anxiety coming along for the ride. Well and truly in the back seat, of course.

The seeds of this book were planted when together we created our online Parenting Anxious Kids course. While researching this course we learned the full extent of the current childhood anxiety challenge and we also grew to understand that there is a great deal parents and teachers can do to assist kids to better manage anxiety. We owe a debt of gratitude to the wonderful Sophie Ambrose from Penguin Random House for sharing our vision of making a meaningful difference in the lives of anxious kids, and for getting fully behind this book from the beginning.

We are grateful to the Australian and international experts who generously shared their time and expertise with us during our interviews for the online course and the book. Each conversation reinforced for us the essential knowledge parents of anxious kids need, and the importance of this knowledge being shared in an accessible way. We'd like to express our thanks to Child and Adolescent Psychologist Dr Chris McCurry. We're in awe of the dedication you have to applying Acceptance and Commitment Therapy to support anxious kids to flourish, and we're grateful for the generous way you shared your time, expertise and anxiety management tools with us. We owe a debt of gratitude to Associate Professor Craig Hassed for showing us how mindfulness impacts on kids' mental and physical health in such profound ways. We were privileged to spend time with Professor Lena Sanci, who showed us the special role that general practitioners play in the lives of anxious kids and their parents. We thank all the other experts who shared their wisdom and experience with us in the course of our research.

We are especially grateful to Russ Harris. The way you bring Acceptance and Commitment Therapy to life with warmth, humour and clarity was the beacon we needed when writing this book. We're grateful for the influence you have on our work and your practical suggestions upon reading the manuscript.

To our awesome team at Penguin Random House: especially Rosie Pearce and Meaghan Amor, we thank you for editing, proofing, typesetting and all of the incredibly hard work that goes behind the scenes to bring a book to life.

Thanks to the wonderful team at Parenting Ideas for your encouragement, your professionalism and for recognising from the beginning the intrinsic worth of this book.

Last but not least, a heartfelt thanks to our families for not only putting up with our frequent writing absences, but for your input when called upon and for wholeheartedly sharing our journeys in the weird world of the expert writer and speaker.

Michael and Jodi